Malignant

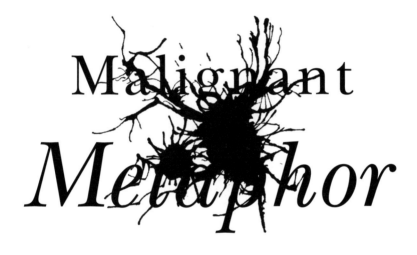

Metaphor

Malignant *Metaphor*

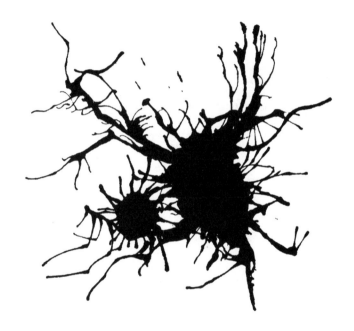

Confronting Cancer Myths

Alanna Mitchell

ECW Press

Published by ECW Press
665 Gerrard Street East, Toronto, Ontario, Canada M4M 1Y2
416-694-3348 / info@ecwpress.com

Library and Archives Canada Cataloguing in Publication

Mitchell, Alanna, author
Malignant metaphor : confronting cancer myths / Alanna Mitchell.

Includes bibliographical references.
Issued in print and electronic formats.
ISBN 978-1-77041-268-2 (bound)
ISBN 978-1-77090-796-6 (pdf) | ISBN 978-1-77090-797-3 (html)

1. Cancer—Popular works. 2. Cancer—Treatment—Popular works. I. Title.

RC263.M58 2015   616.99'4   C2015-902765-9
C2015-902766-7

Editor for the press: Susan Renouf
Type: Rachel Ironstone
Printed and bound in Canada by Friesens: 5   4   3   2   1

The publication of *Malignant Metaphor* has been generously supported by the
Canada Council for the Arts, which last year invested $157 million to bring the arts
to Canadians throughout the country. We acknowledge the support of the Ontario
Arts Council (OAC), an agency of the Government of Ontario, which last year
funded 1,793 individual artists and 1,076 organizations in 232 communities
across Ontario, for a total of $52.1 million. We also acknowledge the financial
support of the Government of Canada through the Canada Book Fund for our
publishing activities, and the contribution of the Government of Ontario through
the Ontario Book Publishing Tax Credit and the Ontario Media Development
Corporation.

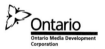

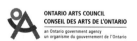

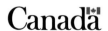

To those dancing with cancer

Table of Contents

❦

Introduction
Inevitable, Preventable and Deserved?

I started writing this book because cancer barged into my life. It was always in the background, pouncing on friends and acquaintances, but then it hit closer. First, my beloved brother-in-law, John, got it. Then, my 21-year-old daughter, Calista, was diagnosed and the quest to understand cancer became even more personal.

I am a journalist who writes about science and medicine, and John asked me to help him learn more about the disease. But I would have done it anyway because I needed to understand more about how this terrible disease was threatening the lives of people I love. And beyond that, I needed to get to the bottom of why the idea of cancer filled me with a sense of powerlessness and dread, in a way that other potentially fatal illnesses do not.

I've spent much of my professional life focused on things that seem unknowable in order to demystify and elucidate them. I think of it as democratizing knowledge. The question I always ask myself is: if we were to take this slice of history and look back at it in 100 years, what would we see that we can't see now? That sense has underpinned my writing on environmental issues, including climate change and ocean acidification. So, when it comes to cancer, what are the stories that we can't yet see? How does cancer show up in our cultural flesh? What meaning courses below the surface, beyond the crushing reality that cancer is one of the biggest killers in the rich parts of the world — the biggest in Canada and the United Kingdom and second after heart disease in the U.S.?

Like so many other important modern phenomena, cancer's contemporary cultural meaning is often shrouded, occluded, even taboo. We come at it obliquely, I think, often not knowing ourselves what we make of it. These subtexts are subtle, unacknowledged, unparsed, like those that have informed racism or sexism or homophobia or xenophobia in human history. Susan Sontag, the American essayist who wrote *Illness as Metaphor* (1978) and then *AIDS and Its Metaphors* (1989) and who died of cancer, argues that we create fantasies about the diseases we understand poorly, lurid metaphors that inhabit the landscape of the "kingdom of the ill."

As I've dug into that landscape, following Sontag's lead from nearly 40 years ago, I've come to believe that cancer suffers from a disease bigotry that shows itself in the stories we tell each other about it, and that it intrudes into our lives in ways we may not recognize.

Those stories are multipronged, like cancer itself. They are not the same for everyone. I have a friend, David, whose lover of 33 years died just 16 days after discovering he had pancreatic cancer. Compared to surviving the institutionalized prejudice of being gay in the North America of the 1970s and 1980s and later watching friends fall ill and die of HIV/AIDS, cancer doesn't bear much of a stigma for David. And today many in the medical profession who treat cancer patients are solemn but not judgmental; it is mainly a disease to be treated. The most recent time I had a breast cancer scare, the surgeon — a lovely, merry man evincing not a shred of pity — asked me a single question: did anyone in my family have breast cancer? When I told him that my mother's paternal aunt had it in her 80s, he looked off into the distance for a moment and then smiled broadly as he said, "I'm not going to hold that against you!" No probing questions about my lifestyle or frame of mind, or darkest secrets, or history of child-bearing and breast-feeding. It was such a relief.

But in general, cancer has a powerful, deadly hold over the collective imagination, far greater than even *its* impressive killing power merits. Our society's overwhelming metaphor of cancer — the meaning it bears within itself — is malignant.

Cancer carries a fearsome stigma for many who get it, as several recent studies show. Those diagnosed feel disqualified from society, shunned. One study catalogs patients whose friends refuse to use the word "cancer," as if it is a jinx or a threat even to utter the syllables. They say friends refuse to see them until they're declared "cancer-free." One described feeling as though she was wearing a leper's bell. Another said people crossed the street to avoid coming in contact with her. A British study published in 2005 found that rather than fear of cancer waning over the years, as scientific knowledge grows and survival rates lengthen, it has remained the same. The British charity Cancer Research U.K. reports that cancer is the number-one fear for the British public, ahead of debt, crime and losing a job. It's a similar picture in Australia.

And some doctors, nurses and other caregivers are just as infused with this powerful imagery as anyone else. When asked to draw pictures of patients who had cancer and AIDS, they drew incomplete outlines, often with internal organs hanging out, writes the Australian poet Cathy Altmann in a cultural critique of cancer. The patients had no hair, no gender, no context. It was as if they had been wholly defiled, their very selves disrupted. Drawings of heart patients by the same medical practitioners, by contrast, were highly detailed, personalized, sometimes even shown with clothing. Heart disease didn't strip the patients of their identity; they just had a problem with their hearts.

I reckon it has come to this: we fear that cancer is three irreconcilable things all at once — inevitable, preventable and deserved. Logically, we know it can't be all three. If it's inevitable, how can it also be preventable, for one thing? If it's preventable, why does a baby get it, or those who lived virtuously their whole lives? If it's deserved, why do some good people get it and some evil people dodge it? Yet that unnamed triumvirate permeates much of the public discourse about cancer, both spoken and unspoken.

When I started excavating our cancer culture, I found many signs of our illogical, impossible belief system, fears buried deep. Let me give you a few examples.

Inevitable: A few years ago when my son, Nick, had just started university — he was in one of those chemistry classes so packed that some of the nearly 2,000 students were sitting in the aisles — his professor wanted to drive home the pervasiveness, the implacability of cancer. Look at the person on your right, he instructed the students. And then look to your left. One of the three of you will die of cancer. Even the cockiest of the students conjured up images of an inevitable mass die-off of the young.

In fact, what the professor ought to have said is that one in three of those brilliant young people will live long enough and healthily enough — dodging infections, accidents and hereditary diseases — to die of cancer. United Kingdom statistics show, for example, that nearly 80 per cent of people who died of cancer between 2010 and 2012 were senior citizens and half of them were 75 or older. Cancer is mainly a disease of the old, not the inevitable plague of the young and healthy. The vast majority of us could bop along pretty safely until we are senior citizens without worrying too much about cancer, unless we smoke.

Preventable: When the child of a close friend was diagnosed with a rare, fatal soft-tissue cancer that had spread to her lungs, everyone who knew her said, "But she's been a vegetarian from birth, eating only organic foods. She's a wizard at soccer and an accomplished dancer. How could this happen?" It seemed impossible to us that such a healthy lifestyle had not been able to prevent her illness. The real story is that her cancer was just random, just terrible luck. Perhaps a quirk of the genetic coding that she was born with. It wasn't her fault and likely couldn't have been prevented by any means whatsoever.

Deserved: A friend was sitting cross-legged in my living room one evening, recently diagnosed with stage 0 breast cancer, some dangerous cells confined to a milk duct that put her at risk for developing invasive cancer. She'd had surgery and had put herself on a strict diet, shunning sugar, wine, flour, wheat and processed foods — among much else — in a bid to prevent more cancer cells from forming. She was keeping her diagnosis to herself, she said. She'd made the mistake of telling an acquaintance about it only to have the woman fix her with a steely glare and demand, "Who have you not forgiven?" Another friend was recently sitting at my dining room table eating warmed-over pasta for lunch. He'd just been diagnosed with prostate cancer. Shoulders slumped, he said his friends were telling him he had gotten cancer because he hadn't had enough sex.

This cultural gloss on cancer, this malignant metaphor, sows immense, widespread blame, shame and fear onto those who are already ill, often fighting for their lives. It spreads to their loved ones and, by osmosis, to a whole society stricken at the thought of getting the disease. Sontag notes that cancer "arouses thoroughly old-fashioned kinds of dread," and that it is felt to be "morally, if not literally, contagious."

Let me delve more deeply into the trope of culpability or deservedness, which is tightly linked to the idea that cancer is preventable: cancer has come to be interpreted as a billboard for the sufferer's secret sins. You did something awful and now you've been found out. Like the transgressors of the Middle Ages who feared an eternity in hell for a single misstep or mis-thought against the teachings of an inflexible church, many people now cleave tightly to a lifestyle code of conduct to forestall a cancer diagnosis, or believe that they should.

This take on cancer reminds me of a contemporary Inquisition: one heretical thought, one unorthodox deed — that urge to sit on the couch after dinner watching a show rather than go on a healthful power walk, or that steak and frites you scarfed down the other evening — and you're done for, outed. The very cells of your body will rat on you, proving the diagnosis of iniquity through the spilling of their inner secrets. And then, like those suspected apostates of old, you'll have to undergo the tortures of mutilation, poisoning, burning, possible social shunning and maybe painful death, in the name of saving not your eternal soul, but your mortal coil. The craze for self-improvement has become resolutely physical rather than spiritual in today's mainstream.

It's even worse than that, when you come right down to it. Apart from tobacco, which is a first-rate carcinogen, and a few environmental substances such as asbestos and soot and several viruses such as human papillomavirus (HPV), it's hard to know precisely what to avoid. That unforgiving code of conduct we're supposed to follow is frequently not based on excellent science. It's suggestive and incomplete and uncertain. And its directives shift with the wind, or with the latest study. That means that even if you could follow all the latest anti-cancer rules to the letter, you'd have to be constantly vigilant, tracking the newest admonitions on lifestyle, the adjurations of nutritionists and television personalities and health columnists and health agencies.

One example. I was just looking at *Science Daily*, a handy site that aggregates news from respectable academic journals and universities. It contains a raft of recent studies on the effects of chemical compounds in red wine, which explain that those compounds can help make prostate and skin cancer cells more susceptible to radiation treatment, stop breast cancer cells from growing and maybe even prevent breast and prostate cancer. But if you google "red wine carcinogen," you get lists of recent news stories telling you explicitly that wine will give you cancer, and linking to government health advisories from around the world that tell you about other studies saying the same thing. Cancer Research U.K. reports, "There is no doubt that alcohol can cause seven types of cancer," and says that 3,100 cases of breast cancer a year in the U.K. are "linked to alcohol."

The oncologist Elaine Schattner, writing about the issue in the *Atlantic*, remarks, "For years now, we — women who've had breast cancer and fear its recurrence, or who are simply at risk, or who are in the throes of it, still — have been pummeled by reports about what we should and shouldn't eat or drink or do. A friend who's had breast cancer complains she can't have a glass of wine without her husband glancing over her shoulder. At family gatherings, her father looks her way, sternly, if she sips from a tall stemmed glass."

The subtext to the adjurations: cancer is preventable, so if you get it, it's because you've done something wrong. But in fact, even if lifestyle choices are linked to getting cancer — a big if unless you're talking about tobacco — it's only a link, not a cause. And if lifestyle choices are linked to getting cancer, they would have to be repeated actions, accumulated over years, if not decades.

The U.S.-based organization Stand Up to Cancer, known as SU2C, which is so tuned into the modern zeitgeist that it hosts a yearly fundraiser featuring the A-list of Hollywood, beats the preventability drum, too, encouraging people to avoid cancer by sticking to their New Year's resolutions to lose weight, quit drinking alcohol and exercise more, spend more time with family and less with electronics and generally enjoy life more.

SU2C, whose funding is administered through the American Association for Cancer Research, is veering past preventability and straight into culpability. It links to a news story in the *Telegraph* reporting a 2008 Israeli study that explains that being happy could cut your chance of breast cancer and that experiencing traumatic events such as divorce or bereavement can increase that chance. The study, whose results have been questioned by other researchers, concluded that unhappy young women ought to be considered an "at risk" group for breast cancer. In other words, if you're happy, you run less risk of getting cancer.

This is cancer shaming, writ large.

Those diagnosed with cancer could be forgiven for tearing their shirts off and beating themselves with sticks in penance. But the truth is that we don't know that much about how we get most of the 200 different types of cancer. Some exceptions are tobacco, directly responsible for about 30 per cent of cancer deaths in Canada and the U.S., and genetic makeup, which is not well understood and is linked to several cancers, including some types of breast and ovarian cancer.

So, what happens once the degenerate cell morphs into the inevitable, preventable and deserved diagnosis of cancer? Well, despite the protestations of sites such as SU2C, cures for each of the 200 types of cancer are not within reach, although they seem closer. In fact, the cancer metaphor ramps up once a diagnosis is made, to that of valiant, dutiful warrior. If you fight hard enough and give yourself over to yet another set of rules and protocols set up by the medical establishment, you stand the best chance of beating the disease, pushing back the "terrorist" of cancer, as SU2C calls it. It's as if cancer really is the war that the oncological fundraising machine and almost every single cancer obituary has invoked.

But the truth is that the route to longer living with cancer, much less cancer-free living, is not always clear; it's a whole vexed and murky odyssey that even oncologists acknowledge is experimental much of the time. The reality is that today, most of those who get cancer will die of it eventually, perhaps having gained a few more years in the wake of obedient treatment, notwithstanding a few beautiful exceptions that include cures for testicular cancer and some leukemias and lymphomas.

The cancer metaphor is flourishing. It is a powerful shorthand that influences behavior, before the diagnosis and after. As the linguists George Lakoff and Mark Johnson say in their book *Metaphors We Live By*, "We have found that metaphor . . . is pervasive in everyday life, not just in thought but in action." Today, cancer's metaphor affects how our society spends its energy and money. It affects what we expect, how we see ourselves, our future and our society.

To me, the metaphor coalesces in the recent phenomenon of "previvors." These are people who have surgery

— often mastectomies — because they fear they might get cancer. There are two types of previvors. Some have a serious and heightened genetic risk of developing cancer.

But people in the second group don't have this predisposition. They choose surgery over possible diagnosis, suggesting they're more afraid of the diagnosis than the disease. In fact, the proportion of American women choosing to have both breasts removed when only one had cancer rose by more than 1000 per cent in the 10 years ending in 2007, according to an analysis of America's massive national cancer database. A separate study found that the extra surgery did little to lengthen the women's lives: it offered just a 1 per cent benefit among those who did not have a genetic risk to start with.

Peggy Orenstein, a breast cancer survivor and journalist writing about the phenomenon in the *New York Times Magazine*, quotes Todd Tuttle, the author of several studies on the needless double-mastectomy phenomenon, who calls it a "mastectomy craze" and confesses that he's worried there's "overawareness" about breast cancer. "Women are petrified," he told Orenstein.

I understand the fear. As Orenstein writes, the fear is warranted. My question is whether *that much* fear is warranted. How does that fear seep through other parts of our lives, in ways not captured by the stark numbers contained in a comprehensive national database about double mastectomies? My question is whether the shame and guilt are reasonable. How do they invisibly influence our society?

Why is the dread so pervasive? I wonder whether some of that dread could be punctured if we understood cancer better. Sontag calls this task the liberation from the disease metaphor. I call it unlocking the science from the academic journals and the operating rooms and releasing it into the public's hands, on the principle that knowledge is its own power. We fear most what we don't yet understand.

What follows is the story of how I stumbled into learning more about cancer, how that led me to dive into figuring out what cancer really is, parse its hidden cultural meaning and, I hope, by telling you the tale, strip a little of the dread away from it.

Chapter 1
Pandora's Jar:
Disease as Punishment

I had been waiting for days to make this phone call, cloistered in Canada's northern wilderness at an aboriginal
healing circle, almost as removed from the modern world
as it was possible to be.

It was the middle of June, when the boreal forest is at its
most beguiling and I, in my role as a journalist, had joined
the others by low-flying float plane, marveling at my bird's-
eye view of this untouched part of the planet. The rivers were
bright blue from up there, meandering crazily through the
trees. Lakes — thousands of them — were by turns as round
as eggs or sprawled loose-limbed over the landscape.

The woods were like a carefully clipped green tufted
rug, except where fire had struck. I could imagine the

fire's mad progress, leaping from treetop to treetop, leaving some alone, charring others cruelly. It was hard to find a pattern.

At the healing circle itself, we had only rough cabins and tents, set in a small clearing excised from the woods. It was overrun with scrubby wild roses, demure pink flowers low to the ground, so different from the sturdy, showy ones we buy in the city.

And we had the stories of the harrowed First Nations people gathered in the embrace of the wide healing teepee, listening to the shamans tell the secret cosmology of how their people and their lands had come to be. It was a step toward recovering faith in the power of these ancestral lands, in their peoples' ways, in themselves. Poignant, tentative triumphs.

Through it all, I was thinking about my husband's beloved eldest brother, John Patterson. He'd already had two diagnoses of cancer, one unrelated to the other. The first, 15 months earlier, in his prostate. Bad enough, and he took to lifting his hand to his forehead in the shape of a "C," like a cipher of shame. His urologist had swiftly excised both gland and tumor, and he had been briefly cancer-free.

The second diagnosis was far scarier. This time it was melanoma, the most lethal type of skin cancer and one of the trickiest and least curable cancers. Now, as I flew north on assignment, we were waiting to hear whether it had spread to his lymph nodes. A no meant that he had a good chance of long life. A yes was the kiss of death.

Finally, the healing circle finished. The float plane returned to pick me up for the first leg of the journey back, and I found myself in the living room of a leader of the Poplar River First Nation, 400 kilometers north of Winnipeg, Manitoba, eyeing the first telephone I'd seen in nearly a week.

The news was catastrophic. The cancer had spread. John had only a 60 per cent chance of being alive in five years.

THE MORAL FORCE OF ILLNESS

It's taken me a while to understand why the news hit me so hard. It wasn't just the unsparing prognosis, although that was part of it. I had already lost two close acquaintances to melanoma in their 50s: my husband's closest friend from childhood and the mother of my son's best friend, whose grisly deterioration over three years I had witnessed.

It wasn't just that I felt helpless so far away in that Ojibway village of 1,200, four hours by road from Winnipeg — if there had been a road.

The more I thought about my extreme grief, the more I realized it had to do with that "C" John had made on his forehead. Cancer means more than the obvious threat to life. But what? And why? Standing in that stranger's living room, straddling the ancient and the modern ways, tears streaming down my face, I know now that I had begun a quest to find out.

Because I am a classics major and studied medieval Latin literature, I started there, delving into the long history of how humans have endowed illness with cultural meaning, even moral force. In the Western literary tradition, you could say it started with the ancient Greek writer Hesiod and his tale of Pandora. The myth says that Pandora was the first human woman, fashioned out of clay in order to punish all humanity and further smite Prometheus, who had humiliated the king-god Zeus by stealing his fire and giving it to humans. Prometheus's fate was to be strapped to a pillar with an immortal liver. Every day, an eagle swooped by and ate out the liver. Every night, it grew back. Gruesome. But not punishment enough for Zeus. He arranges for the sly-speaking Pandora to be offered to Prometheus's brother and when the brother accepts her, she opens a large jar and lets loose on humans an eternity of disease and pain, a counterbalance to the comfort of fire. Disease is the ultimate punishment from the gods.

Homer takes up the trope in the first book of his masterwork *The Iliad*, when the god Apollo, angry at the treatment of one of his priests, sends a deadly plague to the Greek army camping out at Troy. And the writers of the Old Testament describe pandemics as retribution against those who persecuted the Jews, notes the medieval scholar Norman Cantor in his book *In the Wake of the Plague*. The Egyptians endured 10 plagues until the pharaoh let Moses and his people go to seek the promised land.

For as long as humans have written words, we have

portrayed disease as an indictment of character, proof of secret sin or as punishment by some unseen but powerful force. At times, it's the result of the transgressions of an individual; at times, illness affects the individual as a symbol of the wickedness of a whole community. Always implicit is the fear that illness is a sign of something wrong with society itself, a flaw made visible. Illness is about both guilt and blame.

On the surface, this symbol-making was a way of explaining why things happened, part of attempting to understand the universe. So, the ancients imagined that earthquakes struck because the sea god Poseidon, displeased at the actions of humans, thumped the ground with his trident. But it was also a way for society to take a modest amount of control over something that would otherwise be seen as random. They recast it as a social phenomenon, making it the physical match to the leading psychological angst of the day. If only people were good enough, the disease — or the earthquake — would not strike.

Europeans clearly understood the Black Death of the 14th century as the wages of sin, retribution from a wrathful God. Also known as the bubonic plague, it killed an estimated 100 million, wiping out as much as 75 per cent of the population in some regions. In my front hall, I have a framed replica of a fresco from a Berlin church of that period showing the dance of death: pope and emperor, cardinal and king, merchant, abbot, hermit, peasant, maiden, youth and babe. None was spared. All were transgressors.

The attempts to expiate sin and dodge the disease during that period sometimes took shocking form. The religious adherents, the Flagellants, grew to tens of thousands, their numbers rising in lockstep with the dying, traveling from village to village, publicly flaying themselves to atone for sin until the blood ran freely from their wounds.

The plagues continued into the 17th century, successively wiping out great swathes of the European population. London, with its citizens packed so conveniently together, lost a quarter of its population during each wave. Shakespeare's plays, such a reflection of the mood of his time, use the word "plague" 91 times and position it as the epoch's main terror. ("Cancer" didn't have that resonance then. He uses the word only to refer to the constellation, while using "canker," which mainly means a plant-eating worm but can also refer to corruption, just 14 times.)

Leprosy, now also known as Hansen's disease, has been cause for codified social shunning for thousands of years, not because it is a great killer or highly contagious, but because it is a sign of ritual impurity that shows up in extreme disfigurement of the face and limbs. The Bible tells tales of those affected with leprosy-like disease because they had done such things as killing another or disobeying a godly order. Through the Middle Ages, sufferers were confined to leper colonies and forced to wear bells that would announce their proximity to the pure. Even today, India has 1,000 leper colonies.

Tuberculosis was another disease the Western world

used to freight with myth and symbol, as Sontag explains in *Illness as Metaphor*. Responsible for a quarter of all European deaths in the 19th century, it was seen as evidence of one's moral weakness. People wasted away because they lacked ambition or were sensitive romantics with unfulfilled souls or because they simply wanted to be sick. The cure: bucking up.

Then came the Spanish flu of 1918, seen as a vicious extension of the First World War, proof that civilization itself was falling apart. Relentless, it killed as many as 130 million innocents and sickened half a billion, which was then more than a quarter of the world's population. The risks of infection mirrored the risks of an uncertain world, riven by drought, financial collapse and war.

Later that century, it was HIV/AIDS that bore the heavy weight of multiple mythologies, Sontag writes in the 1989 book *AIDS and Its Metaphors*. It was personal punishment for having sex, or having a certain type of sex, or being sexually adventuresome, or even being politically open-minded, she writes. I remember seeing a crude poster in the office of a senior editor of a newspaper where I worked in the late 1980s indicating that to rid the world of AIDS, all you had to do was rid the world of gays.

But all these are fantasy stories. In fact, now we know that earthquakes happen when tectonic plates far beneath the Earth's surface rub together or pull apart, not because a god is angry at man's misdeeds. The bubonic plague was caused by *Yersinia pestis*, a bacteria spread from rats to fleas to humans, infecting humans' lymph systems and causing the horrific black buboes under the arms and around the groin. Leprosy is caused by bacteria that affect the nervous system; tuberculosis comes from bacteria that affect the lungs; Spanish flu was viral; and HIV/AIDS is a tiny, fragile, spherical virus that attacks the immune system and is sometimes spread by sexual activity. Each of these had the power to terrify not just for its killing power — leprosy is not horribly contagious and is considered a chronic disease rather than a quickly fatal one — but because we didn't understand how or why it killed or how it could be rendered benign. Each disease was laden with meaning about the moral correctness of the sick and society.

Today, and for the past half-century, the fiend is cancer.

Nonchalant about the Hydra

John hadn't been worried about the mole on his flank. He showed it to my husband Jim, his youngest brother, the night before he went to the doctor about it. Nestled just below his ribcage on the right, it bore short, dark, rounded tentacles, like a stunted Hydra, the mythic Greek beast that grew two heads for every one hacked off. He had it removed the day after he turned 66 and we had dinner together that night to celebrate the birthday — pasta with red sauce and a big salad. He was in a little discomfort, but said the dermatologist had been confident the mole was clinically boring.

He and his wife, Thea Patterson, were packed and ready to leave the next day for Kenya to check in on a philanthropic project they had started in a Maasai village. The project, born when John had sat under the shade of a baobab tree near the Serengeti with the village's male elders a couple of years before, was aimed at testing every single person in the remote and sprawling Maasai village of 9,500 for HIV/AIDS.

The elders had the unusual idea that if routine testing could remove the stigma of the disease, then people who had it would know they had it, could get treatment and could avoid passing it on. It was revolutionary. No one had tried it before anywhere in Africa, as far as health officials knew, and certainly not among the Maasai, who are outside the mainstream medical system and disproportionately susceptible to getting the virus because of their sexual customs.

Present a challenge and John rises to it. I have known him for more than a decade. He's one of those people whose energy is like a tornado: it draws you in whether you try to resist or not. Invite him into your home and he will naturally take a seat at the head of your table. He never has a small plan; he only has plans that will change the world for the better, that are regionally and continentally and sometimes globally replicable. "Replicability" is a catchword for him. And some of his projects so far have achieved it.

Ordained as a United Church minister like his father, he spent just a few years as a small-town pastor in Ontario with

Thea, a schoolteacher, before realizing that his future was substantially further reaching. He joined an international non-profit organization based in Chicago, the Institute of Cultural Affairs, took a vow of poverty and then set off to India to help some of the planet's poorest figure out how to build their communities in ways that other communities could learn from. Replicability.

In the midst of that, he realized that Asians were in a startling, ahead-of-the-curve boom in information technology know-how, and that he could match Indian brain power with North American need. He and two friends started a company to knit the two together, and named it Kanbay, a riff on the melding of "Canada" and "Bombay." Several years and many investors later, it was listed on the NASDAQ public stock exchange and in 2007 sold lock, stock and barrel to Capgemini for US$1.25 billion, of which John got a small but worthy share. Thirty-two years after he left Canada, John returned, the twice-blessed first-born son: holy and rich. And still devoted to helping others.

The night he had the mole removed, he was actually more worried about the aftermath of his prostate cancer surgery. The surgery had successfully eradicated the cancer, but John had had life-threatening side effects that had preoccupied him for more than a year. Scar tissue had formed around the suturing of his urethra, four times blocking it and preventing his bladder from emptying. Four times, he'd had emergency surgery to reopen the stricture, and seven times, he'd had the stricture physically stretched, an excruciating ordeal performed without anesthetic. Now, to prevent a reoccurrence, he had to insert a sterile catheter into his bladder every day in hopes that the scar tissue would eventually stop growing and leave a permanent opening of a reasonable size.

Going to Africa with that kind of apparatus was tricky, and he'd put off the trip for months. But he was antsy to set foot on Kenyan soil again and see how the HIV/AIDS project was doing and how well the villagers had transferred it to another nearby Maasai village. So he'd persuaded a doctor to go with him as a volunteer, just in case there were complications for him.

She was with him a week after our pasta dinner when he got the first batch of bad news, by cell phone in Nairobi. The mole was melanoma. Not only that, but it was ferociously deep and the dermatologist who had excised it for the biopsy had not gotten it all out. The doctor on the other end of the phone was sorry, but could John please come back to Canada right away?

DEEP INSIDE THE CELL

Just as ancient diviners used to slice open the guts of animals to try to read the future in their entrails, modern medical prophets peer into the molecular structure of a one-cell-thick slice of cancerous tumor to foretell a patient's lifespan. By looking at the secret inner life of a cell — its shape, structure, general orderliness and molecular oddness — they can tell whether the cell is cancerous and how determined it is to spread. Checking distant points from the original site of the cancer — such as lymph nodes — can determine whether it has already figured out how to spread.

What goes on inside that cell to create the phenomenon of cancer is pretty straightforward. That sole cell, just one out of the body's 10 trillion, goes rogue and the immune system doesn't catch it. Going rogue means that a few pieces of the cell's genetic instruction book — which is usually a precise and predictable sequence of pairs of molecules — get messed up. Sometimes little pieces go missing, or extra bits show up, or some get out of order. Think of a favorite chunk of a Shakespearean play whose words are not where they should be: "To not or be to not, that is the answer . . ."

That sort of mix-up is common. Our cells are replacing themselves all the time — probably millions every minute we're alive — and things get mucked up so regularly that each cell has a repair kit built into it with several tools to fix different types of errors. Usually, the repair kit niftily cuts out the misaligned code and replaces it with the correct one. One of the first things the repair kit does is make sure the cell can't reproduce itself with any errors. If the cell detects unfixable errors, it's programmed to commit suicide, no questions asked. Cells are usually dutiful that way.

But a cancerous cell's genetic coding goes wonky in particularly odd and specific ways that bypass the repair system and don't always let the cell kill itself. The altered coding ends up changing what the cells are capable of doing, in effect giving it different messages about what it is for. Those changes mean that a cancer cell can do three main things normal cells don't do: clone itself and evolve endlessly, make itself a blood supply and travel around. Unless the immune system stops that cell in its tracks, this adds up to a cell that reproduces so fast it makes tumors, then creates a blood supply to feed the tumors, and then sends emissary cells through the lymph system or the blood to other parts of the body to do the same thing all over again. That movement is called metastasis, which literally means a rooted thing that begins to move around. So when you hear of someone who has a tumor in his liver because he has colon cancer, it means that he has a mass made up of a single debauched colon cell that has romped through his body to his liver, reproduced itself like crazy and made a tumor. It's not cancer of a liver cell; it's colon cancer in the liver. And it's usually those metastases that kill rather than the original tumor. If the cancer is contained at the original site, it's usually a whole lot less deadly. Metastatic tumors affect vital organs, and when they're big enough, they shut them down. That's cancer's killing mechanism.

The cell's immortality is its secret weapon. While cancer cells can still self-destruct, they clone themselves more quickly than they kill themselves off. As they clone, their genetic machinery accumulates more and more errors, diverting more and more of the cell's energy into the unstoppable drive to grow.

It's a classic, short-term parasitic play: the parasite feeds mercilessly off the host until the host itself dies, finally killing the parasite, too.

Getting Ready to Move

John's single cancerous skin cell had made an unusually big tumor, I can see from reading the pathologist's description of it in the report I have here in front of me. Not only did it grow up from the surface in its tentacles, but it also burrowed deep into the layers of his skin. Generally speaking, the thicker the melanoma, the more chance it has of having spread. And the cells were strange. Even the pathologist who was looking at them under the microscope called them "very bizarre."

Not only that, but the melanoma cells had ulcerated, meaning they had broken through the covering layer of skin. As well, peered at under the microscope, the clones of that one cancerous skin cell were showing signs of high mitosis, meaning they were briskly making new versions of themselves. Both ulceration and high mitosis are signs that a cancer is preparing to move. Of the three things the pathologist can see under the microscope to gauge a cancer's travel-readiness, John's cells had all three: depth, ulceration and a lot of active reproduction.

Even writing this now, sorrow, anxiety and a sense of

fatality overwhelm me. It's as if cancer is everywhere, inescapable for people we care about and even for ourselves. Today it's hot outside — in the 30s Celsius (the 80s to 90s Fahrenheit) — and I'm in a short-sleeved top. My arms are covered in moles, and I've been examining them periodically over the past hours as I've been writing, comparing them to pictures of cancerous moles on medical websites. I can almost imagine the chromosomal mutations taking place invisibly, deep in the guts of one of my cells, warping the cell's intention, cajoling it into thinking it can live forever. Writing about cancer — and reading about it — is terrifying. I can see how our society, convinced that we can control so many aspects of our lives, would make the mystery and randomness of cancer our bogeyman, our metaphor of failure.

FAITH PLUS CYNICISM

When John got back to Canada, surgeons immediately operated again, removing a wide swath of skin around and underneath the original mole and taking out two lymph nodes nearest the mole to see if the cancer was on the move. That biopsy was the one I was waiting to hear about at the northern healing center in Manitoba. If the cancer had spread to the nodes, it meant that renegade cell had executed its dangerous ability to travel.

Both nodes had cancer. And that immediately catapulted the melanoma to the deadly stage IIIb. Stage I is considered an early form and frequently curable. Stage IV is the most serious and means the cancer has traveled far from the original site and into vital organs. It's almost always swiftly deadly. John's staging meant the medical soothsayers who were reading his future gave him a 60 per cent chance of being alive after five years.

And they had nothing to offer him. They considered a few things, such as treatment with interferon, which boosts the immune system to try to attack the cancer cells. But it has not been shown to prolong the life of someone with melanoma by much and it can steal months of those you've got left by making you desperately ill. Plus, John had contracted hepatitis during his stay in India and interferon could resurrect the hepatitis. So that was out. Another reason to thank India, John figured.

He'd had a CT scan of his upper body — a series of x-rays taken from different angles and then fed through a computer program that converts them into detailed three-dimensional slabs, something like being able to see a single slice of bread out of an uncut loaf — and it showed no big tumors in distant parts of him.

Should he have the lymph nodes under his right arm removed, some of which could be cancerous and provide a possible vector for the cells to other parts of the body? The doctors were agnostic. It was a purely personal decision and they couldn't say whether it would benefit him or not. What about eating vast quantities of cruciferous and leafy vegetables, and cutting out sugar and alcohol, and exercising rigorously, and sticking to organics, and adhering to all the other maxims the anti-cancer lifestyle gurus were always advocating? Wouldn't that help keep the cancer at bay?

Nothing would make a scrap of difference, the oncologist replied. It was all too late. But, she added helpfully, when the metastasized tumors inevitably showed up and got too large and painful to bear, John could come back and go under the knife again.

That's really when I became involved. I had been watching from afar until then, worrying along with everyone else in the big, warm extended Patterson clan that I had married into.

The prostate cancer had been one thing. But John had taken the best medical advice he could get, and we all just backed him up. In fact, a critical part of his healing from prostate cancer was his strong personal relationship with his urologist, that he believed in him, despite all the complications that followed the surgery. Shortly after he became his patient, John had scored the urologist's home number and personal email and he wasn't shy about using them. John had built his company by asking people for things.

But this melanoma was a different beast altogether. The disease was life threatening and he couldn't rely on a traditional medical team to take things in hand or give coherent advice. John knew there were other specialists and other alternatives out there, but he had no way of getting at them or figuring out whether they could help. He and Thea were still in the nightmare fog of diagnosis.

39

What treatments were legitimate, which ones might be and which could they ignore? They just didn't know the system. So he asked me to help navigate the world of science and medicine — in effect, to be his cancer broker.

It was an odd pairing. He, the man of faith and action. I, a science journalist, which means I am a professional skeptic and a perennial observer from the sidelines. But while I have no medical training, I can read science and my antennae are finely attuned to nonsense. And I knew I needed to be involved. I'd been dreaming about John every night. Richly detailed, vivid dreams. Sometimes he was in a huge feather bed swathed in thick white linens and I was watching over him. Sometimes, he was almost two-dimensional, part of a pastiche of color, the vibrant browns and reds and purples and burnished golds of illuminated medieval manuscripts that I was trying desperately to read. I would wake deeply troubled, frequently in tears.

So together, we began to explore the untested horizons of cancer research. The aims were to see if we could separate his diagnosis from all the fear and dread that infuse cancer, and to see if we could write a different ending for his story. Like so much medical research over the centuries, this journey, it turns out, would need both faith and science. And while I thought I was the one who would be teaching John, in the end, it was my horizons which were broadened as he taught me what it takes to deal with this harrowing threat to life.

Chapter 2
The Sisters of Fate:
Is Cancer Inevitable?

People have been trying to find remedies for cancer since at least the time the Egyptian pyramids were being built, with varying degrees of intensity. A papyrus describing medical practices from that era describes ancient healers trying to destroy tumors with heated tools and oils. By the first century of the common era, medicinal herbs and botanicals were all the rage. By the second century, it was bloodletting, enemas and induced vomiting, followed, in the 11th century, by arsenical unguents.

Other cures over the ages sound like a sadistic nursery rhyme of mangled animals: boar's tooth, fox's lung, rasped ivory, goat's dung, tortoise's liver, crow's feet, a list offered by the physician Siddhartha Mukherjee in his 2010 Pulitzer

Prize–winning book *The Emperor of All Maladies: A Biography of Cancer.* Some remedies were wishful thinking, or pure guesswork or, sometimes, profiteering. Mukherjee notes that in the 17th century, the price of an anti-cancer salve made from crab eyes went for the mind-boggling sum of five shillings a pound, the equivalent of about $2,000 today.

But what all these have in common is an elusive quest — somehow to forestall death from the roving, degenerate cancer cell.

None of them worked. Until the middle of the 20th century, when the current cancer metaphor emerged and cancer was cast as the ultimate modern plague, doctors had little to offer but frank experimentation. People who got diagnosed with cancer usually died of it quite quickly despite any medical interventions (or sometimes because of them), because doctors understood only incompletely how cancer works. But those early cures took immense imagination, just as some of the modern medical treatments have done. They tried to get to the heart of what cancer is and how it works.

The bloodletting, enemas and emetics revolved around Galen's theory (derived from the early Greek physician Hippocrates, and now discredited) that people got sick when their four fluids or humors — red, white, yellow and black — were out of whack. Letting fluids loose was supposed to help restore order. Presumably the pricey crab-eye paste was a bid to treat like with like, the basis of homeopathy: "cancer" is the Latin for "crab."

The race for the enchanted cure is not very different today. John found that out quickly when he defied one of the cancer metaphor's greatest weapons: he refused to feel ashamed of his diagnosis. He was afraid, but he figured that the more people who knew of his cancer, the more great ideas he would be exposed to for dealing with it. And since John had lived and worked in many parts of the world and visited most of the others, every single surefire cure from one side of the globe to the other ended up in his inbox. He was inundated.

There was the secret potion brewed by an old man in rural Tanzania that would absolutely cure any illness of any sort, cancer included. People were lined up at his doorstep for miles, John's informant averred. There was the super-heating of the body — hyperthermia — in a spate of private German clinics, guaranteed to kill off cancer cells with no ill effects, and magnetic-field therapy offered at the same time to boost the immune system. There were avowals that the cure for cancer depended on daily coffee enemas — shades of Galen — and diets consisting exclusively of pureed raw organic vegetables. Or the assurances that prayer alone had healed many. Or straight goji berries. Or curcumin by the tablespoonful. Or mistletoe extract injections. Or dozens of others. It was bewildering — and overwhelming.

But despite the seeming inevitability of the diagnosis, John and Thea were determined to outwit the prognosis he was given. Without traditional medical help, except routine monitoring, they began to focus on making sure that John was among the 60 per cent with his type of the disease who would still be alive five years after his diagnosis.

While other family and friends tried to barricade John and Thea from the onslaught and took over some of their day-to-day tasks — my husband, Jim, shouldered much of John's volunteer work — I began to run interference on the cancer advice he was getting. I researched the ones that showed any hint of promise, rejecting most of them as too unscientific, too little proven. It often felt as though we were thrust back into medieval times, with people hawking favorite faith cures — crab eyes, anyone? — with absolute certainty they would work and tearful accusations if you didn't at least *try*.

The people who recommended the remedies had a powerful need for them to work. I got that. But the sheer credulity and superstition of it drove me crazy. I am a science journalist, and my whole life has been about sifting through data points and trying to figure out an objective truth, or at least a likelihood. These "cures" were coming in thick and fast without a tittle of evidence that they might work, except the assertion that someone, somewhere might have benefited. They were frequently written so much like traveling circus huckster pitches that I expected to see a flowing cape, magic wand and a top hat, right next to the barrel head where you slap down your money: "Step right on up and see the plucky yoga teacher with metastasized breast cancer who came back from the brink of death with this special diet! And you can, too!"

I wanted charts, numbers, trend lines, pathology reports, comparative scans, randomized blind tests. I wanted, like John, replicability, but not the social type he longed for. I wanted the scientific type. If something really works, you have to be able to produce the same results in more than one person, more than one time, using precisely the same methods. To me, one person's experience does not make a cure.

John was far more open. For him, the important part of any process was to assess the qualities of the people he talked to, understand their points of view, decide for a range of reasons what was most likely to help, and then simply believe in it. Faith, or at least semi-rational risk-taking, was an important part of his process. If traditional medical researchers had given him options to pursue, he would have taken them. But when they couldn't offer him a single thing, he looked to alternative medicines and pushed me to research them.

"There are elements of big mystery to all this, you know," he told me, rather pleased, one day when we were having lentil soup together in a Middle Eastern restaurant.

To Cut or Not To Cut?

As I look back now, I realize that part of the fascination of watching him was his attempt to suss out who the new authority in his life was. He is the son of a minister and open to being dutiful. Before, when he dealt with prostate cancer, he had followed the urgings of his urologist and, peripherally, the formal medical establishment. He hadn't needed to question it too much. It had worked pretty well the few times he'd been sick in his life. Now, he was off those moorings.

But he was used to fluid ideas of authority. I think he relished them. Plus, he was used to throwing himself fully into whatever he did. Born toward the end of the Second World War in 1944, he eschewed the sex, drugs and rock 'n' roll scene of the 1960s. The next thing to a child prodigy, he'd finished high school at 16 and gone to his father's college, Victoria, at his father's university, Toronto, and ended up studying his father's specialty, the ministry, and finally being ordained in his father's Protestant denomination, the United Church of Canada. His first preacher's job had been to take care of a couple of congregations in rural Ontario, much like the charges his father had had, driving madly from one church to another on a Sunday morning, giving sermons and blessing the believers.

That's when he rebelled. He joined the avant-garde Institute of Cultural Affairs, established by people who were disillusioned by institutional Christianity, and hied off to India. Eventually, he became one of the main authority figures in "The Order," as adherents called the institute. And eventually, he withdrew from the Order and made a fortune for himself and many others by working within the authority of the markets.

Now, there was a void. The doctors had all but abandoned him when he needed them most. He needed to find a new team. Like everything else he'd turned his hand to over the years, he threw himself at it with every ounce of energy at his disposal and urged the rest of us along in the cause.

First question: should he have the lymph nodes under his right arm removed? I was astonished that there isn't a protocol on this. I had assumed that if the cancer were stage X, then taking out the remaining lymph nodes was either recommended or not and the surgeon would have the studies to prove it. But that was not the case. It seemed to be just a toss of the dice. John's surgeon was willing to remove his lymph nodes, but couldn't vouch for any benefits.

So I began to read up on the lymph system. It's made of thin tubing running through the body and connecting to some blood vessels, making it a critical part of the immune system and of the blood circulation system. It's akin to a bank for the body's clear blood plasma. Lymph nodes are little bean-shaped disease-fighting factories made to trap cancer cells and bacteria. They gather in clumps in the neck, groin and underarms and deep in your trunk.

I scoured the literature for studies that examined John's situation and compared having the operation to not having it. John had already had what are known as sentinel lymph nodes removed; those are the guards at the gate, the first ones to filter lymph fluid draining from around the original mole. Surgeons inject a little radioactive material

47

and then some blue dye into the skin around the site and follow it to see where it first collects. That's the sentinel, supposed to alert the rest of the immune system army that an enemy is attacking. John had had two sentinel nodes removed. Both contained small clusters of cancer.

Even that surgery is under dispute, although it's usually recommended when the original melanoma is deep, as John's was. But to remove all the lymph nodes in the area is outright controversial. One school of thought has it that if the cancer has already spread to part of the lymph system, it makes sense to get rid of the rest of the nodes in the same area. That's both to remove cancer if it's there, but also to remove a conduit to vital organs for cancer cells that might arrive there. Other surgeons say it's not clear the operation increases the lifespan, so why put the patient through major surgery with side effects that include pain, numbness and swelling, not to mention the financial cost of the operation, either to the patient or to the medical system?

John was torn. His older sister, Barbara Pipher, a nurse and therapist, and the only one in the Patterson family with formal medical training, told him of patients she had known whose arms had been perennially swollen after the operation, and of lengthy, painful recoveries. She wasn't sure it was worth it and was urging him to look at alternative cancer treatments.

The question of whether to cut or not to cut has bedeviled cancer treatments for millennia, as Mukherjee recounts in *The Emperor of All Maladies*. Sometimes, there was an obvious hard lump that a surgeon wanted to have a go at. But early surgeons, in Galen's time and right through to the Enlightenment, usually avoided surgery. In part, that's because they had no effective anesthetic to numb the pain and no antibiotics to treat infections from the surgery. Instead, they tried what passed then for a holistic approach, getting the humors in alignment through bloodlettings and so forth. One of the earliest sites for cancer surgery, however, was the breast, partly because its tumors are relatively easy to get to. The Yale University oncologist Rose Papac notes that early Roman period records exist describing mastectomies.

In his 2002 book *Bathsheba's Breast: Women, Cancer and History*, James Olson tells the ghastly, unusually well documented story of Anne of Austria, wife of Louis XIII of France and mother of Louis XIV, who developed breast cancer in the 17th century. Doctors did not operate, partly because it was revolutionary to do so then, but also because the original tumor was so vast by the time they saw it that they felt it would be futile. Instead they performed the usual bleedings, daily enemas and induced vomiting to cure her humors. But because she was the queen mother, doctors arrived from all Europe to try their pet cures on her, including a paste of belladonna and burned lime over the tumor site, and later a poultice of arsenic on the ulcerating tumors on her breast and underarm. Every day from August 1665 to January 1666, the doctor "took a knife to Anne's breast, carving away dead, necrotic flesh, stopping only when he reached living tissue — normal or malignant," Olson writes. She finally told them to stop and died that month.

In the 16th and 17th centuries, surgeons experimented with a primitive form of mastectomy using fire and acid to remove the breast and leather bindings to cover the wound, Mukherjee reports. By the late 19th century, under instruction from the renowned American surgeon William Stewart Halsted, they were routinely performing so-called "radical" mastectomies that took out healthy lymph nodes in the arm, neck and chest, along with great masses of healthy muscles, in addition to all the breast tissue, no matter how tiny the original lump. The operations became more and more extreme. In some cases, they amputated healthy shoulders and arms and removed ribs and collarbones. Pictures and drawings of the operations look like diagrams for beef butchery. When I come across them in books, I have to close my eyes and turn the page.

The aim of the extreme mastectomy was to eradicate all the cancer cells in the area, to dig deep and "uproot" the disease as if it were a plant with subterranean root systems. In fact, the word "radical" comes from the Latin *radix*, meaning "root." But, as Mukherjee writes, the long-term survival rate of breast-cancer patients treated in this way depended not on the extent of surgery, but on whether the cancer had stayed put by the time the operation began. If it had spread, no amount of excising of healthy bones or lymph nodes or muscle helped prevent death. It wasn't, in the end, how widespread the surgery was, but rather whether the renegade cell had figured out how to travel.

But until nearly the middle of the 20th century, doctors didn't know that invisible cancer cells colonized other parts of the body through the lymph and blood systems, that cancer was fatal precisely because it roamed far away from the original site. Perhaps, those early surgeons had reasoned, it spread locally through muscle and bone. So the theory of taking out as much healthy tissue as possible over as wide an area as possible soon spread to cancers of the cervix and stomach and then to others, sparing, luckily, the prostate.

Eventually, there was a backlash, both among surgeons and among statisticians who were crunching longevity numbers and finding little benefit from extreme surgeries. Patients, particularly breast-cancer patients, felt disfigured. Today, radical surgeries are far less common — the exception is in the previvor movement and the new rush to double mastectomies when only one breast has cancer. Many radical surgeries are even frowned upon unless proven necessary, both for the sake of the patient and for the sake of saving money. And that led to John's dilemma.

THE HOLY GRAIL OF HEALTH

We were booked to go on holiday at a spa the weekend he had to make his decision about the lymph surgery — John, Thea, Jim and I. It was a luxury spa far above Jim's and my pay grade. But Jim was eager to help John, whatever the cost, and we felt John was more apt to show up at the spa on this momentous weekend if we went, too. John's news had shaken the whole family. We had had a sobering meeting of the Patterson clan, more than a dozen of us around the board room table of David, the second brother, a financial wizard on Toronto's Bay Street. Along with brainstorming about how to help John, we had all pledged, heads slightly lowered, to lead healthier lives: lose weight and de-stress.

So, despite my misgivings that we were submitting to the dictates of the metaphor, we found ourselves wrapped in plush white robes at the Grail Springs spa near Bancroft, Ontario, lined up for five self-indulgent days of lovingly prepared low-calorie organic meals, massages, mineral soaks and a host of other body- and mind-purging rituals, with the offer — here's Galen again — of colonic irrigation, which is the modern way of saying enemas.

Many of our fellow spa-mates were fans of colonics, billed as the unerring way to gain "mental clarity and a strong sense of well-being." You could tell who they were because they invariably came to meals in their white bathrobes, toting ampules of chlorophyll and acidophilus tablets, the spa's prescription for building up proper intestinal bacteria post-treatment. They would line them up beside their plates of vegan food, a badge of honor for those healthfully clean bowels.

The place had a medieval gloss, as the name suggests, complete with a Chalice Lake, the Camelot Trail and the claim that deposits of healing crystals, magnetically potent minerals and "holy" waters on the property would encourage the place's healing powers. I couldn't help comparing it to the bare-bones First Nations healing lodge I had been to a month earlier in northern Manitoba.

I had sworn off even the vegan fare, opting instead for a three-day-long juice cleanse, meaning I was on a liquid diet of fresh vegetable and fruit juices. I'm not sure why. It's funny how the lens of scientific rigor slips when you're desperate to help someone and fearful of the implications of your own dodgy living habits and growing girth. And it was only for three days.

We were immersed in ritual body adoration, if not acceptance, our flesh anointed with oils, all our toxins reputedly excreted through our pores or trundled away by our bodies' lymphatic tubes even now massaged into obedience by the therapists. The Holy Grail, I guess, was to change, becoming thinner, healthier, more disciplined, perhaps more like the people who ran the spa.

And smaller breasted, apparently. As one of the therapists was giving me an excruciating reflexology session — pressing hard on every tender point along the edges of the feet and toes — she confided that one of the male massage therapists always complained about treating women with big breasts because he found them unaesthetic. Plus, he had to prop up their shoulders with rolled towels when they lay on their stomachs. I flinched and crossed my arms over my breasts. What would he say to treating someone with cancer? I asked. He wouldn't touch a cancer patient with a ten-foot pole, she replied. The bad energetics would simply ruin him.

In the meantime, John had decided to get a second opinion and had made an appointment to consult a team at Memorial Sloan-Kettering Cancer Center in New York City, the world's oldest and largest private cancer clinic. He was flying there shortly after he left the spa, just days before he was tentatively booked to have the lymph surgery back in Toronto.

In between skin-brushing sessions and fortifying mud drinks, we gathered in John and Thea's sumptuous room, plotting strategy, accompanied by just a touch of forbidden cabernet sauvignon wine. Asceticism only takes you so far. Our goal was to set down what questions John should ask the experts in New York, including whether or not he should go ahead with the surgery. As well, John had a sheaf of academic papers from alternative medical journals for me to read, including one on the controversial use of intravenous vitamin C to treat cancer, and several on injectable mistletoe extract supplements.

John wanted more than just a surgical decision. He was looking for another set of doctors to tell his future from the inner workings of that one delinquent cell and all its clones. So we set about writing up lists of questions in bold markers on two large sheets of paper. Had the New York doctor ever had a patient with this kind of melanoma whose cancer didn't metastasize to other parts of the body?

Had he ever had one who had lived a long, healthy life?

I still had one chunk of my brain mired in the literature from earlier eras, thinking about the bodies of all those women whose breasts and muscles and bones had been carved off them, with little anesthetic and no antibiotics. It's hard not to take those stories personally. I was reliving my last mammogram, the one that found something, my own small cancer scare. The hospital had called me back and asked me to come in for more tests.

The day of my appointment, I examined my bare breasts in front of the mirror, feeling for a lump, looking for a pucker or the telltale patch of orange-peel-textured skin. I have big dense breasts (the spa's massage therapist would have been horrified) and have had benign and worrisome cysts in them since my early 20s when I first started regular attendance at breast cancer clinics. These days, my palms barely cover my nipple area and it's hard to look at all the breast tissue thoroughly. I could see nothing.

The acrid smell of my own fear overpowered me. I was worried not so much that I might have cancer as what the diagnosis would say about me, that it would divulge my secret failings. Finally, I looked myself straight in the eyes and told myself, "This could be the last day of your life that you think you're cancer free." I felt like throwing up.

In the end, it was all histrionics. The anomaly was a large, liquid-filled cyst in the left breast. Not cancer. Not dangerous. It would subside on its own as I moved through menopause.

My fear was bigger than the risk merited. Bigger because the metaphor was in full bloom all around me. Why was I so afraid? Again, I sought the wisdom of history. Cancer wasn't always seen as "the ultimate illness," that Mukherjee talks about. For most of the thousands of years it's been around, it's been seen as a sporadic blight rather than judgment on a whole populace. Anne of Austria told her confidante that she felt humiliated that she had breast cancer and thought it was the hand of God punishing her because she had been vain through her life about her good looks, Olson recounts. So it was personal retribution for her sin of vanity. But breast cancer was uncommon, and cancer as a whole was relatively rare in the 17th century. It wasn't seen as the societal scourge that, say, common infections were then, in an age without antibiotics.

This is when I first began to conclude that cancer's resonance today lies in our perception that it is inevitable, preventable and deserved, all at the same time, an impossibility that takes your head and spins it around. It's an unholy trinity. Inevitable because it feels as though everyone has it or is going to get it. It's as though the sisters of fate have woven into our genetic fabric a cell destined to kill us. Preventable because the underlying social discourse tells us if we do all the right things, we will dodge the bullet. And deserved because we somehow think if we get it, it's because we've done something wrong. The kicker is that at the same time, cancer is cast as the "quintessential product of modernity," as Mukherjee writes. So the messages are that we're going to get it, it will be our fault and it's a byproduct of this civilization we've made. In a way, we're all complicit in every diagnosis.

THE INESCAPABLE DISEASE?

I decided to tackle the first of this triumvirate. Is cancer really inevitable? Are most of us really fated to get this terrible disease?

It certainly feels as though it touches everyone, that we all know someone who has it. And no question, there is much more cancer in absolute terms today than there has ever been in the history of humanity. The World Health Organization (WHO) says 14 million people around the world were diagnosed with cancer in 2012, of the planet's 7 billion. And it's growing. In two decades, it will be about 22 million. The message implies that cancer is inescapable.

But actually, there are two main reasons there's so much more cancer today than there was a few decades, or even centuries ago. First, there are more people on the planet than ever before, so the number of cases grows along with that. But second, so many more people are old, and cancer is largely a disease of the old. In fact, the number of people over 60 nearly tripled between 1950 and 2000 and it's set to more than triple again by 2050. That would represent an unprecedented rise from 205 million older people to nearly 2 billion in just 50 years. And that means a lot more cancer. It goes back to all those molecular machinations in the body's cells. The longer a person is alive, the more time the cell's inner workings have to make cumulative batches of errors that aren't fixed. So the older you are, the more likely you are to get cancer. The older the average age of the population is, the more cancer there will be in the world.

But here's the shocker. If you adjust for age and population growth, these days there's actually about the same chance or even less of getting cancer and dying from it in the U.S. and Canada, along with other wealthy countries. Here's the bottom line from a landmark study on global trends in cancer by Ahmedin Jemal and others, published in *Cancer Epidemiology, Biomarkers & Prevention* in 2010: ". . . cancer rates in general are decreasing in the United States and many western countries." This is not at all the headline we get at nearly every turn.

In fact, we hear the opposite. The Stand Up to Cancer (SU2C) website declares that cancer is a "worldwide epidemic," that a new cancer is diagnosed every 30 seconds in the U.S., and that every three minutes, another two Americans will die from cancer. The underlying metaphor makes cancer sound like a ticking bomb, an endless march of death from a foe we should all be working hard to fight, because it's going to get us or our loved ones next, like a stealth assassin we could forestall if only we were vigilant enough. The language is an object lesson in dread, in doom.

But the statistics actually describe a different, less fearful trend that's rarely talked about: less cancer pouncing, and when it does, patients living longer after treatment. Take Canada as an example of where the numbers are in the richest countries. Age-adjusted analysis from the Canadian Cancer Society and Statistics Canada finds that the incidence of breast cancer rose from 1982 until the early 1990s and has leveled off since. The death rate from breast cancer, the most common one for Canadian women, is the lowest it's been since 1950. Stomach cancer rates for both men and women are about half today what they were in the early 1980s, and death rates from stomach cancer are at a third.

Lung cancer, the big one for Canadian men, has been on the wane for men since the mid-1980s, both in how often it hits and in how often it kills. It's the opposite for Canadian women, but projections are that the rates of lung cancer for women will also start to fall now that more of them are abandoning tobacco. Cancers of the cervix, larynx and mouth are on a downward trend. Prostate cancer is on a modest increase, after spikes in 1993 and 2001 as prostate antigen blood tests were pushed. Death from it has taken a sharp decline. In fact, in Canada, two of the few cancers on the rise affect the liver and the thyroid. The causes for thyroid cancer are unclear. Liver cancer rates are on the upswing because of an increase in the incidence of hepatitis B and C.

It's a different picture in eastern Europe and many of the poorer countries, where smoking, cancer-causing infectious diseases and lack of physical activity — a problem because it can lead to obesity, which is a risk factor for cancer — are becoming more common and therefore cancer is, too, even among younger citizens. All in all, in the rich parts of the world, about 30 per cent of men and 22 per cent of women will develop cancer before they turn 75, according to a study published in 2011. So that's slightly less than one in three men and a little more than one in five women. The risk for those in poorer countries is a little more than half of that in the rich countries: 17 per cent for men and 14 per cent for women.

It's a lot of cancer, but this is not the picture of inevitability. In most countries, cancer isn't even the biggest killer. (Canada and the U.K. are exceptions, partly because they do so well in treating heart disease, leaving people alive long enough to get cancer. One has to die of something, in the end.) In 2012, the latest year for global figures, just less than 15 per cent of the world's 56 million deaths were from cancer, totaling 8.2 million. The biggest known contributor to those 8.2 million was tobacco smoking, which accounted for one in five of them. That same year, more than twice as many people (17.5 million) died from cardiovascular disease, which is rarely considered a global epidemic, as from cancer. And one and a half times as many (12.8 million) died from communicable diseases, mother and baby deaths and deaths from malnutrition. Death from injuries, both unintentional, like car accidents, and planned, like suicide and war, came in at another 5.1 million, about two-thirds as many people as died from cancer.

Public health authorities are frank about the fact that

the reason cancer ranks as high as it does on the global death list today is because so many other diseases that used to kill us are now treatable and, in some cases, preventable. We just don't hear about it. That's why there's less cancer in poorer countries: it's because there's more chance of dying from something else first. Antibiotics, which were unknown until the 1940s, have saved millions of lives. Routine immunizations, which ramped up in the last half of the 20th century, have saved many millions of people from getting sick. Smallpox alone killed between 300 million and 500 million in the 20th century and is now uncommon because of vaccines.

A glance at the statistics for the U.S. aptly describes the shifts in killers across the rich part of the world. In 1900, when the average lifespan was 49, the biggest killers in the U.S. were pneumonia and the flu. Cancer ranked eighth on the list that year with only 3 per cent of the deaths. By 1950, when antibiotics were in widespread use, heart disease was by far the biggest killer and cancer was a distant second, with about 15 per cent of the deaths.

By 2013, the latest year for statistics, heart disease was still the biggest killer in the U.S., killing 30 per cent of Americans, and cancer was second, with 22 per cent of the deaths. Flu and pneumonia had fallen to 8th place, with 2 per cent of the deaths, roughly where cancer had been at the turn of the previous century.

And while once, if you got cancer, it was pretty much game over, now in some parts of the world, the death rates for some cancers have been pushed back. That's partly because more cancer is being caught earlier and excised or killed with drugs or radiation before it learns how to travel, and that means it doesn't get the chance to grow deadly tumors in vital organs. If it does metastasize, then cocktails of chemotherapies, which only started to be experimented with in the mid-1960s and which are now the main way of treating advanced cancer, can urge some of them toward remission. Testicular cancer, once almost a guarantee of death, is now considered mainly curable, along with a handful of others, including some blood and lymphatic cancers.

In the United States, the Centers for Disease Control and Prevention reports that in 2013, 163 people died of cancer for every 100,000 in the population, adjusted for age. In 1999, the figure was 200, which means that a smaller proportion of Americans are dying from cancer than once did. And cancer is not as immediately deadly, statistically speaking. In 1975, if you were diagnosed with any kind of cancer, it was a coin toss whether you would be alive in five years — pretty much an even 50–50 split. By 2010, those odds of surviving to five years had increased to 68–32.

The advances are partly an artifact of mashing together of a lot of numbers. The National Institutes of Health (NIH) says that most of the reason that the death toll from cancer has dropped in the U.S. is because the rate of smoking has fallen by nearly half over the same period, rather than solely because of the billions of dollars ploughed into research and treatment.

And are we surrounded by people with cancer? Is it everywhere we look?

The big picture shows that 4.5 per cent of U.S. citizens — or 14.5 million — are living with cancer, and nearly half of them are 70 or older. In Canada, things are counted slightly differently: roughly 2.5 per cent of the population is living with a cancer that was diagnosed within the past decade.

To me, the numbers tell a different story than the cultural messages of predetermination. They tell me that cancer is common but less common than it used to be and somewhat less deadly. But it doesn't feel that way. It feels as though it's our galloping modern plague.

All of this was going on in my head as I sat drinking wine with John, Thea and Jim at the Grail Springs spa. Our list of dozens of questions for the team in New York was done, written in fat marker on vast sheets of newsprint. I had expected John to type them into a Word file and print them out so they'd be neater. But he folded them up and put them in his briefcase. He would take them to Sloan-Kettering just the way they were, he said. He wanted an answer to every last one.

Chapter 3
Billboard for Sin:
The Fables of Disease

As John and Thea flew to New York to try to find out more about how the melanoma would play out in his life, I became obsessed with the stories we weave around how disease comes about. How do they connect to the overwhelming myth that getting cancer is inevitable and that if you get it, it's somehow your fault? It was hard for me to figure it out, so, to get some perspective, I went far away to another culture and then back in time.

A few years ago, I was in Tanzania with John, Thea and Jim to work on an HIV/AIDS prevention project with the iconic Maasai people.

The Maasai roam the scorched, drought-ridden savannah of Tanzania and Kenya, tending the cattle that are still their currency, so tall and so thin that their shins and cheek bones seem to slice open the air they walk through. Many live in their own communities in huts made from thatch and cow dung, apart from other Africans. They cling to a pastoral lifestyle that is harder and harder to maintain as society shifts around them and as the drought leaves their cattle emaciated.

Their lands seem mystical, untouched by time: herds of zebras off in the distance, lions, alert, crouched in waiting. One day, as I drove down a dusty highway, giraffes wandered nonchalantly across the road. The Maasai live near the expanse of the Serengeti and the Olduvai Gorge in the ancient rift in the Earth's crust that is considered humanity's cradle. It still occasionally sets free the fossilized remains of our species' ancestors.

Despite the ancient lore of the land, a modern disease, HIV/AIDS, is spreading among the Maasai, and Tanzanian health officials are worried that it will have uniquely widespread and devastating effects on them. The Maasai custom is for men to have more than one wife at a time — sometimes a dozen or more — and share them with other men. And as the cattle-rearing lifestyle has become tougher, many of the Maasai men have journeyed to towns and cities in recent years for work and have come back home infected with the virus.

But some of the Maasai don't believe that they can get HIV/AIDS, they told me. It's something other Africans get, and it's critical to the Maasai understanding of their role

in society to think they are immune. It means health officials have trouble persuading them to get tested, get treatment or wear condoms to avoid passing the virus on to
sex partners. One community health-care worker I spoke
to told me about a man with advanced AIDS whose family
tried to get a local shaman to heal him by making circles
around his head with a chicken.

The myth-making is not so much about the disease itself
or about shame or even about sex. It's about cosmology:
the larger story about how and why the world works and
where they fit into that world. It doesn't suit them to think
they can be infected the way other people are.

Trying to reshape that myth was the focus of the project
John and Thea helped bring to life in the Kenyan Maasai
community of Il Ngwesi, the one they were visiting when
John got the call that his mole was melanoma. There,
the Maasai elders, more science-minded than many and
alarmed as people from their community wasted away with
AIDS, wanted the whole village educated with the modern
medical understanding of how the disease is spread. It was
a bid to have science infuse myth, for knowledge to triumph over narrative.

They asked John for help to find the money. Then they
gently encouraged everyone in their communities to be
tested so they could prevent future infections. Painstakingly
implemented over several years, the testing has helped
change minds and therefore perhaps behavior. The Maasai
community is trying to spread their new understanding of

how the disease takes hold to other Maasai communities, trying to get others tested and treated so fewer will die. Knowledge, in their case, is life.

Once I could read the Maasai fable, I scanned back through European culture and found it replete with similar myths about disease, many of which were eventually also combatted with knowledge. The example that resonated the most was that of the high rate of death among young, healthy women who got fevers after giving birth in clinics and hospitals. Childbed fever was the most common reason new mothers died in the 18th and 19th centuries and the second most common cause of death of women of child-bearing years, behind tuberculosis. It was characteristic for up to a quarter of new mothers who gave birth in the crowded, unsanitary hospitals to die of puerperal fevers. During some outbreaks, it killed them all. Mothers who gave birth at home or with midwives rather than doctors rarely died of the fevers.

For centuries, physicians thought the illness spread mysteriously through the air from one woman to another. Eventually, a few progressive doctors began to wonder whether it was something more concrete. It was common practice in early hospitals for birth attendants to go directly from autopsies to births, sometimes using the same instruments, wearing the same clothing, often having dissected the corpses of women who had died of childbed fever the day before. Hand washing was frowned upon. It went against doctors' understanding of who they were: it was seen as prudish and ungentlemanly.

In the 1840s, European obstetrician Ignaz Semmelweis, who worked at the Vienna General Hospital in Austria and later at St. Rochus Hospital in Hungary, wondered if there could be a link between the autopsies and the births, sparked by the death of a colleague who died of a fever after cutting himself with a scalpel he had been using during an autopsy. Semmelweis advocated that medical attendants wash their hands with antiseptic soap. Then he totted up the numbers, which showed that the hand washing led to a sharp decline in new mothers' deaths. He was vociferously ridiculed, a "prophet without honor in his time," according to a history of maternal deaths published in the *Journal of the Royal Society of Medicine*. He died in an insane asylum.

By 1879, the French bacteriologist Louis Pasteur, whose method for sterilizing milk still brings him renown, finally showed irrefutably that swabs from women who had the birthing fevers could frequently grow *streptococcus* bacteria in lab cultures. That meant the bacteria were in the bodies of the dead women and that, in turn, suggested that doctors were the carriers of disease rather than just those who cured it. It was a blow to the medical ego. Then microscopes, through which physicians could actually clap eyes on the bacteria, became more common and the germ theory of disease was born. The concept of preventing new mothers' fevers through the use of hand washing, sterilization and antiseptics took hold in the late

1800s. Women's deaths from postpartum fevers are now rare in parts of the world where antibiotics and sterilization techniques are available.

THE MAKING OF A DEBAUCHED CELL

When it comes to cancer, the landscape is also intimate and emotionally freighted. It's a discussion about your body's particular molecular machinery and the fact that your body's survival mechanism is impaired. What made that happen?

The big-picture answer has gone through several philosophical changes over time. By the mid-18th century and the rise of empirical thought, a few doctors began questioning Galen's theory of the humors. They noticed that exposure to chemicals was linked to the high incidence of certain types of cancers. The *British Journal of Industrial Medicine* recounts the story of the London surgeon Percivall Pott, who noticed that a lot of young soot-drenched chimney sweeps were dying from cancer of the scrotum. Originally, those cancers were attributed to sexual depravity, even though some of the young patients had not yet hit puberty. But then a gardener who spread soot on his plants nearly died of a similar, massive tumor engulfing his hand and Pott began to imagine that the soot itself could cause cancer. His case studies in 1775 have been called the first medical description of an occupational cancer.

He wasn't alone. In 1761, Londoner John Hill noticed

that people who used snuff were getting cancers of the nose and by the 1850s, the French physician Étienne-Frédéric Bouisson noted that it was his pipe-smoking patients who were getting lip cancer. These findings were revolutionary, pointing to the idea that some causes of cancer were outside the body instead of nestled inside it, or inside one's mind.

Eventually, Mukherjee explains, that thinking led to the powerful idea that underpinned the U.S.'s heavily financed, heavily marketed war against cancer during the 20th century: all cancers have a single cause, a single mechanism and a single cure. It was the reigning scientific principle, but it was also an effective fundraising slogan. Billions poured into the quest to find that one cause.

More recently, that idea has evolved again. The medical world has begun to see cancer as an umbrella term for about 200 different diseases all triggered by a rapaciously cloning cell. They can look inside the cell to see that different pieces of the cell's genetic instruction book are affected in different ways to make different types of cancer. So while all cancers share similar characteristics — rapidly cloning themselves and not dying off, cloaking themselves from detection by the immune system, traveling and making their own blood supply — different segments of their genetic code mutate in different ways and in different combinations to achieve those ends, cancer by cancer. In fact, even within a single type of cancer in a single body, the cloned cells are continuing to change as they divide.

Now, that thinking has gone even further. Not only do different cancers come about from different genetic aberrations, but the same kind of cancer can also happen from a range of different mutations in the rogue cell. The large Canada-U.K. 2012 METABRIC study (Molecular Taxonomy of Breast Cancer International Consortium), which looked at 2,000 breast tumors, concluded that there are 10 different types of breast cancer, each with its own molecular fingerprint, each needing to be treated differently. Increasingly, the watchword in cancer today is to think of personalized causes, personalized treatments, the opposite of the "one cause, one mechanism and one cure" philosophy that characterized the original war on cancer. This is one reason the refrain of personal blame creeps into the discussion more than ever; since your cancer configuration is personal, your lifestyle must be at fault.

But how do the genes change? This is the fraught question. Sometimes, the propensity is born in you, an inherited disposition you carry within your double helixes that fosters cancerous intent in the cell. These are called the genetic causes of cancer, and researchers are at the very early stages of understanding them. At the moment, they're thought to be responsible for perhaps two or three per cent of cancer cases. Among the best understood cancer-causing genetic mutations are those that affect the BRCA gene, potentially causing breast and ovarian cancer.

The American actor Angelina Jolie, whose mother died of ovarian cancer, astonished the world in 2013 when she announced that she had had a preventative double mastectomy in a bid to cut her likelihood of developing breast cancer to 5 per cent from the 87 per cent she had inherited along with the gene. Two years later, she had surgery to remove her ovaries and fallopian tubes to lessen her chance of developing cancer in those organs. Her move has sparked an upsurge of women — known as the "Jolie effect" — asking to be tested for the BRCA mutations. But few other inherited mutations that can cause cancer are understood as well as that one.

Some infections can lead to cancer, too, an idea that has gone through waves of medical and public controversy. At one time, cancer researchers thought most cancers were viral. Then, they swung against that idea, focusing on other causes. Today, their research shows conclusively that some strains of the human papillomavirus (HPV) are the main cause of cervical cancer and can cause cancers of the throat, vulva, vagina, penis and anus; viral hepatitis B and C can cause liver cancer; and the bacterium *Helicobacter pylori* can lead to stomach ulcers and cancer. Doctors have developed anti-cancer vaccines for some HPV strains and hepatitis B, a huge breakthrough in the prevention of cancer and the first time our species has been able to immunize against any type of cancer.

But the controversies over whether children ought to get the HPV vaccine at 11 or 12, before they become sexually active, have been rampant, particularly in the U.S. and Canada. Some argue that while it might prevent cancer, it might also acknowledge that teens could be sexually active and encourage them to have sex. A few years ago, Michele Bachmann, then a Republican Congresswoman from Minnesota, called the vaccine "dangerous" and implied it can cause mental retardation, claims swiftly rebutted by doctors. But only about a third of the young Americans who ought to be vaccinated against HPV are, and parents are wrestling with the cultural meaning of vaccinating against a sexually transmitted cancer-causing virus. This is not about scientific knowledge, but about beliefs, fears, prejudice.

And then there are the environmental and industrial pollutants, many of them chemical compounds invented in the past several decades by humans to make growing food and other commercial enterprises easier or more efficient or more profitable. Some of those substances — both natural and man-made — have been shown to be capable of altering the genetic code of cells and can lead to cancer. It's one of the reasons the Environmental Protection Agency in the U.S. has set up a whole protocol to scan some new chemicals for their carcinogenic properties and bans them or limits their use if they are cancer-causing. Among the brilliantly effective, proven carcinogenic substances are soot, tobacco, arsenic, asbestos, radiation and some of the byproducts of combustion, including benzene.

But the story may be bigger than that. A 2010 report to U.S. President Barack Obama from the President's Cancer

Panel on reducing cancer risk from the environment says that "the true burden of environmentally induced cancer has been grossly underestimated." It mentioned that of the 80,000 chemicals on the market in the U.S., many in daily use by citizens, only a few hundred have been tested for their cancer-causing properties. That means we're exposed to cocktails of chemicals. Many of them have not been tested for effects they have when they are mixed within the human body, Cynthia de Wit, a professor of environmental science at Stockholm University, told me recently. These may have only tiny effects individually on humans, but we're exposed to so many more of them today over so many decades and in such weird new combinations that it's unknown what they do to our genetic coding.

And a whole new class of manufactured chemicals, the endocrine disruptors, affect the hormone systems of adults and children and are even passed to unborn children, according to scientific analysis published in the 1996 book *Our Stolen Future* by the biologist Theo Colborn and two others. Most are not regulated for those properties, although some, like DDT and the pesticide dieldrin, have been banned from use in some parts of the world. They still show up in astonishingly high concentrations in soil even where they're banned, though. Some of the hormone-affecting chemicals are currently under investigation for increasing cancer risk to parts of the body directly controlled by the hormone system, including the prostate gland, the testes and breasts, among others.

At this point, the bottom line is that ecotoxicologists around the world are worried about the effects of chemical cocktails on the health of humans, but so far few studies are looking at links to cancer. Their actual, rather than estimated, effect on cancer rates is unknown.

The President's Cancer Panel urged Obama to boost research into all the questions raised by chemical contaminants. Panelists said the environmental and chemical causes of cancer have gone "largely unstudied," despite the vast amounts and numbers of new chemicals the human body is exposed to over time. Instead, far more cancer research money has been spent on looking at one's own genetic predispositions and personal habits than on environmental causes.

The suggestion is that it's easier to point the finger at an individual's lifestyle and choices than it is to question a widespread societal system of production and manufacturing. Viewed through the lens of the malignant metaphor, though, it would seem far more helpful to know whether those chemical cocktails actually cause cancer because if they do, we could limit our society's exposure to them through regulations already in place and waiting to be used, such as those of the Environmental Protection Agency. If society has unwittingly created a pool of risk for cancer, society could also eliminate or lessen that risk and correct its mistake.

But if research on chemical exposure and cancer is meager, the idea that emotions or personalities cause cancer has been studied rather intensively for centuries, with more focus in the past several decades. And the working theory has been that your own personality or character flaw causes cancer. That idea is pervasive, just as it was with tuberculosis, leprosy and even the plague. If you were happier or better adjusted, you wouldn't be sick. You are to blame. You deserve to get cancer. This idea underpins much of the mythology, the metaphor that infuses our cultural understanding of cancer.

The medical doctor Paul Rosch, chairman and founder of the American Institute of Stress in New York, has been an influential researcher into the link between mind and disease. In a chapter he wrote in the Sloan-Kettering Institute cancer series book *Cancer, Stress, and Death* published in 1979, Rosch summarizes the history of academic thinking on how your own attitude makes you fatally ill. He says that even very early medical theorists believed that grief or sorrow could cause cancer. Galen, for one, says that melancholy women, those afflicted with too much black bile and therefore sorrowful, are more prone to cancer than other women. Rosch cites the 18th-century English physicians Gendron and Burrows, who say that grief and long-term "uneasy passions of the mind" are responsible for causing cancer. Doctors of the 19th century blamed emotional factors for breast cancer and said sensitive and frustrated married women were more apt to get cervical cancer than those who were neither sensitive nor frustrated, Rosch writes. Later, in the 19th century, the cause for breast and uterine cancer was said to be the loss of a near relative and that, in general, "habitual gloomings of the temper . . . constitute the most powerful cause" of cancer.

By the 20th century, the idea that some people have a "cancer personality" had taken hold, meaning that some people have an emotional, rather than genetic, predisposition for developing cancer. Early theorists pointed to people who were anti-emotional or too rational as prime candidates for cancer, or too extroverted and not neurotic enough, or too prone to suppress negative emotion or who were traumatized by the birth of a sibling.

Rosch cites the 1970 book *Happy People Rarely Get Cancer* by Jerome Rodale, founder of the wildly successful *Prevention* magazine, and the 1977 book *You Can Fight for Your Life: Emotional Factors in the Treatment of Cancer* by the influential American experimental psychologist Lawrence LeShan as examples of works aimed at explaining how attitude influences the course of cancer's progression.

And the Australian poet Cathy Altmann, in her critique of cancer and metaphor, points to the metaphysical U.S. author Louise Hay, whose book *You Can Heal Your Life*, has sold more than 30 million copies and was a bestseller on the *New York Times* list. Hay's point is that we create every illness we have and we can use thoughts and words to cure them, including cancer.

The idea that your attitude controls whether you get cancer and then whether you survive it was so compelling that by the mid-1980s, the clinical psychologist Lydia Temoshok published her theory that there is a Type C (for cancer) personality, characterized by the suppression of emotion, by self-sacrifice, self-blaming and the need not to upset the applecart. Those negative thoughts impaired the immune system or increased inflammation, the suggestion was, meaning the Type C person was more apt to develop cancer and to fail to fight it effectively. Temoshok recommends changing attitudes to heal from cancer.

And it's a similar case with the Australian author Ian Gawler, whose book *You Can Conquer Cancer*, has sold more than a quarter of a million copies and been translated into 14 languages since it was first published in 1984. An updated edition came out in 2012. He, too, says there is a Type C personality, which he says is created by trauma at a young age. Cancer patients are victims, in Gawler's analysis, notes Altmann.

It all leads to the overwhelming sense that the successful cancer survivor is a bold, outspoken and optimistic person who wants to live, writes the Romanian psychologist Diana Tăut in the journal *European Health Psychologist.* Of course, the implication is that the person who dies from cancer is weak, timid and pessimistic.

Ultimately, it's about blaming the patient. Or society itself. One of the themes that courses underneath the idea that individuals are responsible for their own illness

79

is the idea that society is responsible, too. I have the image in my head of a grand communal self-scourging, like the Flagellants of old.

Much of the early work on the causes of cancer points squarely to modern civilization as the culprit. Rosch mentions, among many other references, that Albert Schweitzer, on reaching Gabon in 1913, found no evidence of cancer and that Canadian ethnologist Vilhjalmur Stefansson found no cancer when he first visited the Inuit of the Arctic but did later as the Inuit came into closer contact with non-Native civilization. Stefansson turned his findings into the book *Cancer: Disease of Civilization? An Anthropological and Historical Study*, published in 1960.

Rosch is most impressed by a 1957 book on cancer by Alexander Berglas explaining that cancer almost only affects those who live in modern civilizations and that every living person is "threatened with death from cancer because of our inability to adapt to present day living conditions." Rosch concludes that cancer is a "disease of maladaptation" and suggests tests to identify the depressed in society in order to treat them and prevent their getting cancer.

It sounds compelling, doesn't it? Even though Rosch's work and that of the researchers he quotes are now several decades old, the ideas still infuse some of the medical and, more importantly, the public discussion about cancer. The power of these ideas is abetted by the primeval stories of our species' search for a link between fate and the divine.

Perhaps that's knitted into our genetic code, too. What if you get cancer because you are unhappy or can't cope with modern civilization very well? It's a vision of the survival of the fittest: if you can't handle modern life, cancer will kill you off. There's a rough justice to it, on the surface, and seemingly a cold-blooded evolutionary logic.

It's a narcotic idea because it plugs into all our unknowns about how cancer actually shows up, how that one cell goes rogue, how the body forsakes itself. And then the what-ifs start to creep in. What if it's because I'm not happy enough? What if all this anxiety I have about meeting this deadline right now is going to fatally mutate one of my cells? I keep thinking of Sontag's line in *Illness as Metaphor*: "Theories that diseases are caused by mental states and can be cured by will power are always an index of how much is not understood about the physical terrain of a disease."

The problem is that while the idea may be insanely appealing as a human narrative, there's actually little science to support the finding that sorrow or grief or depression or being emotionally distant or any other personality trait causes cancer. But the idea that your own personality defects can cause cancer is still so pervasive, even among those in the medical profession, that now researchers have begun massive, long-term studies to test it.

One of the most robust of these, published in 2014 in the *British Journal of Cancer* by Markus Jokela and others, is a meta-analysis (a study of studies), pooling information from six huge, multi-year investigations covering nearly

43,000 people, whose average age was about 52, from the U.K., the U.S. and Australia. At the start of the study, none of the 43,000 had cancer, but over an average of five years of follow-up, 2,156 developed the disease. The personality type of each of the original 43,000 was sorted into one of five categories, based on what's known as the Five Factor Model (or "The Big Five"), recognized as the most comprehensive and universal classification of human personality types. The five are known by the acronym OCEAN, which stands for Openness to experience, Conscientiousness, Extraversion, Agreeableness and Neuroticism.

The findings? No type of personality was linked to a higher risk of cancer, or to a higher risk of any specific cancer, or to a greater risk of dying of cancer. And the authors point to several other extensive studies that have similar conclusions. Despite centuries of medical teachings, there is a distinct possibility that the Type C personality does not exist and that your own character flaws don't make a cell go bad.

DEADLY SINS

And then there are the "lifestyle factors" that may trigger or prevent the mutant cell. Here, the research is intensive, almost frenzied.

What is it about how you live your life — what you eat and drink, how much you exercise — that makes you more susceptible to the degenerate cancer cell? Some of the research is driven by this puzzle: people who live in different countries tend to get different types of cancer. For example, the most common type of cancer among Chinese women and men is of the stomach. In the U.S., it's breast cancer for women and prostate cancer for men.

And when immigrants arrive in Western countries, they become as affected by the cancers of their adopted countries as those born there. That's an indication that there is an environmental or perhaps social element affecting which cancers are most common. So there's a rich vein of research to look at why those differences are happening.

But this is also where the narrative of shame creeps in, the overweening story that cancer is the direct result of your personal failings. If you were a good person, you would prevent that deranged mutant cell from taking over your body. The World Health Organization, for example, along with listing the known carcinogenic chemicals and infections such as tobacco and HPV, goes on to say that physical inactivity, diet, alcohol use and being overweight are all implicated in getting cancer.

In fact, it says that more than 30 per cent of cancers globally are preventable, meaning — here's the headline no one wrote — that something less than 70 per cent are not. But it also says 22 per cent of cancers are linked to tobacco use and 1 to 4 per cent are from environmental pollution. That means the WHO is saying that the remaining 4 to 7 per cent of cancers are preventable by avoiding all the other possible causes combined, including such things as radiation, sunlight, infectious agents and your personal habits. How much is the result of personal habits? Unclear. This is very hard stuff to study.

In 2011, British cancer researchers published a landmark study that tried. It examined how 14 "less than optimal" lifestyle and environmental factors might affect cancer: diet, body weight, reproductive history, exercise and several other things, all of which must have been long-standing. So it's not just the bloody sirloin steak you had last night for dinner; it's a lifetime of suboptimal living. The study, published in the *British Journal of Cancer*, concluded that about 43 per cent of cancers in the U.K. are linked to those factors. Like the WHO, the British study pinpoints tobacco use as the biggest risk factor, responsible for more than 19 per cent of cancers, or nearly half of the ones it says are preventable. For men, the next biggest culprits are lack of fruits and vegetables (6.1 per cent of cases), occupational exposure (4.9 per cent) and alcohol consumption (4.6 per cent). For women, it's being too fat (6.9 per cent) followed by infections, mainly sexually transmitted (3.7 per cent).

The study takes pains to explain that it is not saying that all these cancers could actually be prevented, just that lifestyle factors — sometimes several at once — may contribute to the likelihood of getting cancer. The aim, the study says, is to help public health officials figure out which strategies they should focus on first to help curb new cases of cancer.

But, partly because the information is complicated and the message hard to explain, that's not how it gets played in the medical and public discourse and in those sleepless middle-of-the-night sermons to oneself. In this narrative, you could prevent cancer if only you were virtuous or strong-willed enough. And if you get it, it's because you've done something wrong. Cancer is a billboard for your most secret sins, your evil excesses. The truth — how little difference the missed Zumba class and paucity of organic broccoli makes — gets lost.

So if you get mouth or throat or, god forbid, anal cancer, it's because you've had unprotected, untraditional sex — the deadly sin of lust combined with non-conformity. Breast cancer? The lore says it's because you didn't have children, didn't have them early enough, didn't breastfeed them, didn't breastfeed them long enough, drank too much red wine, ate too much fat or a combination of these. In other words, the sin of self-indulgence or perhaps vainglory, like Anne of Austria.

Men who get prostate cancer routinely report being ribbed about having had too little sex, the evil of self-abnegation, or too much, the sin of greed or, perhaps, uxoriousness. (It was one of the common cancers for which the British study found no link to a "less than optimal" lifestyle factor.) People with thyroid cancer hear that their throats are closing up because they've failed to voice their thoughts and emotions, the sin of repression. Bowel cancer is a sure sign of the dreadful moral failing of constipation, unless you call it colorectal cancer, in which case, it's because you're overweight and lazy, thus the sins of gluttony and sloth.

Cervical cancer means you were lustful and had too many sex partners too young and without the use of condoms and spermicidal foam. Melanoma is evidence of the sin of hubris: going into the sun without covering up and believing you would be left unharmed. Esophageal cancer? You're a drinker, a smoker and you have a poor diet. Or else you're fat. Pancreatic cancer? You eat too much.

And the list goes on. Stridently. Jane Cawthorne, a Canadian writer who was diagnosed with Hodgkin's lymphoma, a cancer of the lymph system, in 2004, writes in her essay "The Cure for a Cancer Cliché":

> I once read that if I drank pomegranate-flavored antioxidant martinis, I could have fun and reduce my risk of cancer at the same time. In this version of prevention, if we live right (which is never too different than how we live already) we will not get cancer.
>
> If prevention focuses on individual action, it should come as no surprise that causation does as well. Any failure to take care of ourselves, get enough exercise or eat well becomes a source of blame. . . . Like the warning against a negative attitude, focusing on how people cause their own cancer is a powerful tool to keep us all quiet. We must reap what we sow, pay our karmic debt, live (or die) with the consequences of our actions.

Under the circumstances, we are lucky to get any help at all.

The medical research quest to figure out just what you're doing to cause your cancer is in full bore. Here is a recent smattering of new findings — many of which contradict other studies — courtesy of the science news aggregator *Science Daily*: the more alcohol a young woman drinks before motherhood, the greater her risk of breast cancer; breastfeeding for more than six months helps prevent breast cancer; stress affects whether breast cancer cells can travel to other parts of the body; eating yellow-orange vegetables reduces the risk of invasive bladder cancer in women, but not men; failing to brush and floss regularly can lead to the cancer-causing oral HPV infection; pancreatic cancer can stem from a poor diet; dying from pancreatic cancer is linked to heavy drinking; but drinking four or more cups of coffee a day can forestall the recurrence and spread of prostate cancer.

What's lost in all this is that none of these are absolutes. Each of those personal activities is loosely linked to a higher risk of getting some kinds of cancer, likely in combination with a host of other unknown factors over many years. They're not causes — like tobacco and soot — but potential risk factors, frequently of an unknown potency.

And some of them are not exclusively personal activities. The food most people eat is produced by industrial systems our society has set up. Personal choice is only part of the issue. What of the massive, ingenious advertising push to sell sugar, salt and fat to people, potentially encouraging them to become overweight? What about the systemic use of pesticides to grow food? Does that cause cancer? It's unresolved. What about hormones and other synthetic chemicals in meat? Again, unclear. And there's a financial aspect to this. In the Western world, it costs more to eat more healthily than it does to eat poorly.

The truth is that we don't know all that much so far about exactly what triggers the cell to run amok. And a lot of it may happen for no reason at all, just random mutations in a single cell over time. Yet today, just as it has been through the ages, it seems to be psychologically important to society to come up with reasons for the illnesses. That's borne out by all the maxims about how to live, which show up as a mysterious, ever-changing, contradictory and tyrannical lifestyle code that we must all follow lest we be fated to join the blighted brotherhood of the damned. If only we were pure enough, the sublimated message runs, we could avoid getting cancer. If only we were dutiful, we could spare ourselves and our society the dreadful punishment of cancer.

It's like a new version of the old Christian dictates that told us we must eat fish on Fridays, a mandate so closely followed that scientists can now track the depletion of fish from European rivers and coasts through the centuries to that one rule. It's like the priests who once told people when they could have sex and who with and in what position. Except today, the rules extend past the kitchen and bedroom and into nearly every room in the house and even into the gym. The goal is not saving one's soul, but saving one's body, preventing the plague of cancer.

Cancer as Metaphor

In his 1991 book *Grace and Grit: Spirituality and Healing in the Life and Death of Treya Killam Wilber*, which is about his wife's death from breast cancer at 42, the American philosopher Ken Wilber published passages from a diary she wrote shortly after she was diagnosed:

> Was there some secret death wish here? Had I been too hard on myself, too judgmental and self-critical, such that secret self-hatred caused this? Or had I been too nice, repressing my anger and judgments, so they eventually manifested as this physical symptom? Was I being punished somehow for having been given so much in this life, a family I really enjoyed, intelligence and a good education, attractive looks, and now this fantastically-beyond-belief husband? Was one only allowed so much, so that going beyond triggered adversity of some kind?

To Ken Wilber, her worries illustrate that any disease has two distinct elements. The first is the illness itself, or the physiological process going on in your body. In the case of an ear infection, it's a bacterium or virus that is growing too fast in the inner ear. In the case of cancer, it's a cell that's gone on an unstoppable growth spurt. The second element is what he calls the sickness of a disease, which he defines as the meaning a society gives to it.

He writes,

> And so whenever illness strikes, society is on hand with a huge supply of ready-made meanings and judgments through which the individual seeks to understand his or her sickness. And when that society is in fact ignorant of the true cause of an illness, this ignorance usually breeds fear, which in turn breeds negative judgments about the character of the person unlucky enough to come down with the illness. . . .
>
> Now cancer is a disease, an illness, about which very little is actually known (and there is virtually nothing known about how to cure it). And therefore, cancer is a disease around which an enormous number of myths and stories have grown up. As an illness, cancer is poorly understood. As a sickness, it has assumed awesome proportions. And as difficult as the illness of cancer is, the sickness of cancer is absolutely overwhelming.

What he is saying is that these myths around cancer make up a social construct, not a medical truth. Cancer has become a metaphor, one that is difficult to identify because we're in the throes of it. I think it is driven by an unspoken fear that, like the Black Death of the 14th century, cancer is really about the sins of our society. This is why John made the C on his forehead. This is why the massage therapist at the Grail Springs would have refused to touch John because he has melanoma. This is why Susan Sontag concluded that cancer is "morally contagious."

So what is cancer, viewed through the lens of the public imagination, seen as metaphor?

It's the lethal enemy we create within the microscopic workings of one of our very own cells. It is a fiendish, insatiable, homicidal version of us. It is a remorseless creature determined to grow bigger forever, greedily using up ever more of our most precious resource: the body's energy. It takes and takes until it literally cannot take any more, on a ruthless quest to colonize, to dominate, to bend the other trillions of cells in the body to its perverted will. It refuses to share, taking anything it wants, leaving nothing for others, not caring how many casualties or how much devastation it leaves behind. It respects no boundaries, no natural laws. It never rests, working around the clock on its obsessive vocation of non-stop, exponential growth, enlisting its unthinking clones in the same relentless enterprise. When powerful outside forces invade the body on a mission to kill it off, it changes just enough to outwit them, hiding and biding its time until it can muster more force and take over for good. And once it's finished its rapacious romp through the body, its fatal miscalculation suddenly becomes clear, too late, and it dies, along with you.

We've unleashed the ultimate enemy, the one that will kill us invisibly from within, making manifest the fatal weakness of our system, the proof of our lack of control and foresight.

Because a lot of my writing is about how humans are damaging the life-support systems of the planet, all of this rings a bell. This popular understanding of cancer mirrors the scientific critique of modern society, the one that is so profoundly disturbing to so many of us and that has spawned decades of debates at the highest international levels about pulling back from the brink. So far, these debates have been fruitless and the human load on the planet gets ever nearer the lethal levels that will produce the sixth mass extinction in the history of life on Earth.

According to the science of the planet, humans are the enemy from within, using up too much of the Earth-body's resources, changing the very chemistry of the air and the sea with our uncontrolled burning of fossils, impairing the planet's ability to support us and other creatures. Like cancer cells, our numbers grow exponentially and our effect on the planet does, too. And we're acting mindlessly, parasitically, with little consideration for how it's affecting others, driving vast numbers of plants and animals toward extinction. We're not taking into account whether our descendants can survive in the future. Like cancer cells, we somehow think that we can bypass natural laws. Now scientists are warning us that if we keep on doing what we're doing, the planet may become inhospitable to us within mere decades, like the parasite killing its host. So in some ways, what we're doing is even worse than what

cancer cells are doing because unlike them, we can imagine the consequences.

One reason cancer is so powerfully resonant is that it
is a metaphor for what humans are doing to the planet.
And what humans are doing to the planet is a metaphor
for cancer. They plug into each other, invisibly reinforcing
each other. Our great fear is not that we're at the mercy
of an angry Greek or Roman or medieval god. Our fear is
that society is so flawed we'll exterminate ourselves, and
our actions will have justified it. In other words, we've
somehow given ourselves the idea that cancer, or global
mass extinction, is inevitable, preventable and deserved.
It's a recipe for madness.

SECOND OPINION

As I was grappling with all this, John and Thea were in New
York with a team of experts. By this time, Thea had started
carrying a spiral-bound, lined book with her, taking notes
at all the medical appointments so she and John could
review them later. She gave me copies of her notes written
in her schoolteacher's hand, each letter resting on the line,
each letter carefully formed even though she was taking
her notes on the run. I marvel at the steel she had, sitting so
outwardly calm through those meetings that tried to foretell her husband's future and, in so many ways, her own.
They had just celebrated their 40th wedding anniversary.

John had had the luck to get an appointment with

Daniel Coit, a specialist in cancer surgery who mainly studies melanoma. Specifically, he assesses the future of people who have already had surgery for melanoma, trying to figure out what any remaining melanoma cells mean to do. Melanoma is an uncommon cancer — only 133,000 people around the world had been diagnosed with it that year, 2010 — and Coit is a rare expert in reading its strategy.

Coit developed the technique of mapping sentinel nodes and was one of the promoters of removing the sentinel nodes first and then assessing the need for a full lymph node removal. Before this technique became common, other far more invasive surgeries were routine. He's one of the leaders of Sloan-Kettering's melanoma management team. When John showed up in his office with our big pages of marker-written questions, Coit's eyes lit up and he went through each one with gusto.

John had gone into the meeting in distress. The doctors in Canada had essentially told him to go home and wind up his affairs. They had nothing to offer him and said nothing he did now would affect his lifespan. He was likely to be dead in a few years. They couldn't even recommend whether to remove the remaining lymph nodes on his right side. John describes the whole tenor of his appointments with the Canadian doctors as "funereal." He was frustrated by the impression they gave him that he had no control over whether he lived or died.

Sloan-Kettering couldn't have been more different. The tone was upbeat, relaxed. First off, Coit strongly encouraged John to have the rest of the lymph nodes removed. If it were him, he'd do it, he said. He added that when the sentinel nodes already had cancer — as John's had — about 15 to 20 per cent of patients would have cancer in nodes deeper in the lymph system. If John were among that group, it was worth having the cancerous nodes out. He was not concerned that John would lose the use of his arm, or that he would have trouble healing, calling the surgery a "non-event" for those issues. John, he said, would be playing golf in no time. He recommended physical exams every three months and CT scans every six months to check for lumps. He discouraged John from trying the alternative treatments he was considering, saying there's not enough evidence that they work.

Then came the big questions: had he ever seen a patient with this staging of melanoma whose cancer had *not* spread? Certainly, said Coit. Had he ever had a patient like John who had lived to be 90? Yes, he said. How could John take back control and try to make that happen? The key, Coit said, was to control what John could control: a healthy diet and plenty of exercise.

All of this was completely at odds with what John had heard in Canada. John put it down to individual differences between doctors, pointing out that Coit was a couple of decades older than his Toronto oncologist and clearly had learned the value of equipping his patients with images of possibility and hope. He and Thea breathed a tentative sigh of relief and flew back to Toronto. Two days later, he was on the operating table, having the rest of the lymph nodes under his right arm taken out.

Then the waiting began again. If the biopsy found melanoma cells in none or just one of the nodes, the severity of the cancer remained the same: stage IIIb. If it were in two of the nodes, that would catapult it to stage IIIc. And that would mean his life expectancy had taken a sharp drop: from about a 60 per cent chance of being alive in five years to a 40 per cent chance.

Chapter 4
The Haruspex:
Defying the Dread

We waited nine days to find out if any of the other 11 lymph nodes were cancerous. And it was worth the wait. We got the best possible news: none had any trace of melanoma. The cancer remained at stage IIIb. John's chance of being alive in five years remained at 60 per cent, instead of slipping lower. Cancer plays with your mind so savagely that this time, when we knew that his chances were 60 per cent, the prediction felt like a small victory, rather than the calculus of doom.

And here was the fascinating thing for me, grappling as I was with the cultural evolution of humanity's response to cancer. With no traditional medical options except routine monitoring, John's imagination took flight. All of a sudden, all bets were deliriously off. Rather than letting himself fall permanently into the dread of the cancer diagnosis, he tried to strip it of some of its power, to look at it unblushingly. I found myself mesmerized by his response, taken aback and even puzzled by his newfound sense of freedom.

That's not to say he had no bad moments. He did. I remember a troubling trip to Quebec City shortly after the diagnosis, with him and Thea and Jim. John seemed always to be two steps ahead of us, racing to escape his mortality. He had plans, big plans, and he couldn't let the cancer slow him down.

One of the first things he did was tell everyone he knew that he had cancer. He eschewed shame, blame and self-pity. He never asked himself, "Why me?" Not once. He wasn't really interested in knowing. He wasn't sure how long he had left to live, but he was determined to make it a marvelous ride.

And because all traditional medical methods had now been exhausted, he started to assess alternative therapies. He started looking at his melanoma in a different way than he'd looked at the prostate cancer.

His sister Barbara had heard of the work of Ralph Moss, an American expert in alternative cancer treatments. Moss, who has a Ph.D. in classical literature, once worked as assistant-director of media relations for Sloan-Kettering and now operates a well-respected clearinghouse for information on both conventional and non-conventional cancer treatments offered in several parts of the world. He publishes more than 200 reports, called *Cancer Decisions*, each one tailored to a different type of cancer. Cost: US$297 apiece.

He also publishes occasional papers on emerging cancer topics, such as boosting the immune system, and offers phone consultations for US$500 for the first hour. He bills himself as an impartial middleman for those diagnosed with cancer, perhaps one of the rarest commodities in the multi-billion-dollar industry that has grown up around cancer treatments worldwide. John's brother David became intrigued, bought the report and then both brothers spoke with Moss on the phone.

The message was unabashed hope.

The Moss philosophy is that conventional U.S. and Canadian cancer specialists are blinkered, bound to work only with therapies that are already approved and rigorously tested in North America. That means they unfairly ignore unconventional therapies, including some used routinely in other developed countries, on the grounds that they don't have enough scientific rigor behind them. Within that framework, though, Moss still insists on careful analysis of whatever evidence is there.

Moss's comprehensive reports — the melanoma one John got ran to 442 pages — encompass recommendations on diet, European clinics, traditional therapies, and seemingly every single other folk remedy out there, including coffee enemas, goji berries, Chinese mushrooms, shark cartilage, mistletoe extracts and dozens of others. Moss assesses the latest scientific findings around each of them, trying to help people ford the bewildering torrent of options and crank cures that appear after you've been diagnosed with cancer. Then he puts them all together in a single report and makes recommendations about whether they show promise. You can't help but feel that you're getting a peek at the future, an exhilarating chance to be ahead of the curve.

The reports represent a massive amount of information, some of it quite technical. I wondered how much of it most patients would be able to take in. And I wanted to know whether people who consulted Moss and followed his advice had any different lifespan than those who didn't. It would be a fiendishly difficult experiment to run, containing immense numbers of variables, I know. Did Moss's patients eschew chemotherapy, for example? Did they combine alternative therapies with traditional ones? Were they more prone to alter diet and exercise, or devote time to meditation?

In the long run, I couldn't tell whether it mattered that cancer patients had sought other ways of treating their diseases. For me, this was troubling. Without the rigor, the science, the trials and at least some degree of certainty, how could we know anything about whether the therapies will work? It was still not nearly enough information for me. Taking these therapies was an act of faith, not reason.

John didn't see it that way at all. He treated all the

alternative therapies as a fascinating and deadly important experiment and was eager to explore some of the most promising ones. Four of the unconventional therapies caught his attention. The first was diet. Moss, like Sloan-Kettering's melanoma specialist Daniel Coit, emphasized using a healthy diet and exercise to support what he calls an anti-cancer lifestyle. For Moss, the prescription was organics, organics, organics. The connection between food grown with pesticides and risk of cancer is largely unexplored. A few comprehensive studies suggest that organically grown foods have higher levels of some anti-oxidants than traditionally grown foods. The idea is that plants need to create higher levels of those chemicals in their own cells in order to fight off pests. Other studies show that antioxidants can help prevent some cancers. Organic foods also have lower levels of pesticide residues in them than those grown with synthetic chemicals.

John was already a fan and the idea of buying food that doesn't have residual amounts of pesticides really appealed to him. Less potentially toxic stuff for his body to deal with had to be a good thing, he reckoned. But he lived in a town three hours' drive north of Toronto, where the availability of organic food was not good. So, as an opening gambit, he started making sure that people who drove up to visit him brought organic produce.

Second was injectable mistletoe extract, one of the most widely prescribed anti-cancer medications in use in parts of Europe. John had already been to see a medical doctor in

Chicago, Ross Rentea, who straddles both traditional medicine and naturopathy. Rentea had strongly recommended injecting mistletoe every day. There's some evidence that extracts of a European form of the plant can prolong life if used with traditional therapies, according to an analysis of 49 studies published in 2009 by Thomas Ostermann and others. Studies have found that two compounds in the plant help kill cancer cells, boost the immune system and protect healthy cells. John was keen to start an experiment, so he started injecting himself with mistletoe.

Third was the compound DCA, dichloroacetate, an old drug already approved for use in children who have metabolic problems. Evangelos Michelakis, a researcher at the University of Alberta in Edmonton, had run some tests to see whether DCA could also be effective in killing cancer cells in a test tube by interfering with the cell's metabolism, and had then tried it in lab animals. The result was a headline in the respected *New Scientist* journal saying that the drug could kill most cancers both safely and inexpensively. That got translated into the far sexier headline that Michelakis had found the cheap cure for all cancers, hearkening back to the decades-old dream that there is one cause for cancer, one treatment and one cure. It was the longed-for magic bullet.

Of course, it caused an online stampede, and people ordered the drug without any sense of how much to take, how often. The quest for cures is impassioned, and the quest for cheap cures, especially in the U.S. where some patients spend their life savings on medical treatment and even bankrupt themselves, is unrelenting. Many people, perhaps only months away from death, felt they had literally nothing to lose by trying an experimental drug.

Michelakis was finally forced to publish a disclaimer. DCA is also known to be a carcinogen in lab animals in high dosages, for example. Then he raised $1.5 million privately and ran another test on five patients with advanced brain cancers. The results were encouraging, but the study is tiny. At the moment, research is stalled. That's led to accusations — very common in alternative cancer circles — that because no big company can make big money on this drug, it will never be tested enough for anyone to know whether it really works. Moss's assessment was that DCA shows exciting promise and he predicted that fully funded trials were inevitable and will happen soon. He urged patients to wait until proper trials are conducted before taking the drug on their own.

However, a single clinic in North America was prescribing DCA as an anti-cancer treatment. It was in Toronto.

David thought it was worth examining. I thought it was the equivalent of a Hail Mary pass when none was warranted. John's cancer was at a relatively early stage, with no metastasis to vital organs. This drug was unproven, possibly unnecessary and possibly dangerous. If John ever got to an advanced stage, I could see that it might be worth a try then. Still, John made an appointment with the clinic in Toronto to check things out. It was a bad fit. Even the naturopathic doctor there told him his cancer was too early to be treated with DCA. Plus, John just couldn't see himself being treated there and said he wouldn't do it. His response amazed me. I was discovering that a critical part of how he was approaching this disease was that he needed to bond with the people who were going to be taking care of him. It was an intensely personal, intuitive process.

THE TALE OF THE VITAMIN

Fourth was vitamin C. Like the mistletoe injections, this was a treatment Rentea, the Chicago medical doctor and naturopath, had recommended. Treating cancer with vitamin C has a decades-long, highly controversial history threaded through with legendary battles, big egos and bitter recriminations. It began nearly 50 years ago when the Canadian physician William McCormick started thinking about how vitamin C might affect cancer cells and published a paper on it. The Scottish surgeon Ewan Cameron took the thinking further and used small doses of it on 50 patients who were dying of cancer, then compared their longevity to that of patients elsewhere who were not treated. He was terrifically excited by some early results.

At about the same time, the Nobel Prize–winning chemist Linus Pauling, also a winner of the Nobel Peace Prize, was coming to a new kind of fame by claiming that vitamin C could cure the common cold. So Cameron took his findings on vitamin C and cancer to Pauling and the two of them ran some more tests on patients with advanced cancer. They published their results in two papers — one in 1976 and another in 1978 — saying that 10 grams of vitamin C a day could send cancer into remission and prolong life. Their 1979 book on the topic, *Cancer and Vitamin C*, electrified doctors and the public alike. It was the miracle cure: a simple, cheap treatment using a substance as familiar as the orange juice on your breakfast table. Plus, it had the heft of a double Nobel Prize winner behind it. In the wake of all the excitement, Pauling publicly accused the medical establishment of refusing to embrace his bold new findings.

Researchers at the Mayo Clinic in Minnesota took that at a canter and ran two sets of tests to see if they could replicate his findings. It was a disaster for the proponents of vitamin C. The new studies showed absolutely no effect from using it. For many doctors, the sense of betrayal was huge and the idea that vitamin C could help cancer patients became a running medical joke.

But recently, despite the stigma, a handful of doctors have begun looking at it again. They discovered that vitamin C taken orally doesn't get to nearly as high concentrations in the bloodstream as that dripped straight into the veins. It turns out that the Mayo studies used exclusively oral vitamin C while Pauling's studies used a combination of oral and intravenous. By about 2000, some doctors began investigating vitamin C again, quite tentatively. Some naturopaths, drawn by the early claims and the fact that side effects from using the substance appear to be minimal, had begun prescribing it, too.

Moss was not a big fan. His view was that the treatment showed promise, but he wanted to wait for the results of further clinical tests.

He dropped one new idea into the mix: the emerging field of looking deep within the composition of the blood for the presence of traveling cancer cells. Doctors had long been able to diagnose blood and lymph cancers from looking at blood, but the idea of identifying cancers in other parts of the body just by poking a vein has been a tantalizing dream for decades. Doctors have dubbed it the liquid biopsy, and if it were ever to be reliable, it would mean a blood test could diagnose cancer rather than surgery to remove tissue.

The theory is that as an original tumor cell gets the idea of staking claim to other parts of the body, it will use the lymph or the blood system, or both, to move its clones around. If technology could be precise enough to spot those few colonizers among the great wash of other cells and count them, it might give some idea of the cancer's strategy. Several labs around the world have begun experimenting with tests to do that — including one method that has been approved by U.S. regulators — and Moss thought it might be worth John's while to try one. He wasn't too keen on the one U.S. regulators liked, but instead recommended an outfit in Bayreuth, Germany, run by a husband and wife team, Ulrich and Katharina Pachmann.

CELLS IN THE BLOOD

John's driving goal now was to find a naturopath near his home to administer intravenous vitamin C, which he had decided to try. He was already on a daily pill regimen of fractionated pectin, mushroom extract, goji berries, chia seeds, noni juice, green tea extract and curcumin (derived from turmeric), plus daily injections of mistletoe extract. The naturopath whom Rentea recommended in Toronto was fully booked and couldn't take John on as a patient. So John ended up in the offices of Peter Papadogianis, in Barrie, Ontario, partway between John's home and Toronto.

Papadogianis, a naturopath who also has a Masters degree in pathology and is used to looking inside cells, had been administering intravenous vitamin C for more than a decade, treating hundreds of patients with it. He reckons that he is one of about 100 practitioners in Ontario providing the treatments. He was excited about treating John, who was at a comparatively early stage of cancer and had not had chemotherapy. That meant he was a new kind of patient whose experience might prove clinically important. Replicability.

As well, John was highly motivated to stick to a grueling regime and could pay for regular intravenous treatments at $145 a pop. He had both the money and the grit to be the experiment and had even considered funding research into the efficacy of the vitamin. But John also wanted Papadogianis to draw blood periodically and send the samples to the Pachmann lab in Germany, just to see what they said about the presence of cancer cells in the blood and to track any changes. Papadogianis agreed.

So they began. By the end of October 2010, six months after John had had the mole removed, he'd finished a series of 12 infusions of 50 grams of vitamin C each, fed into a vein in his arm along with sterile water, calcium, magnesium (to help relax the blood vessels), a smattering of all the B vitamins and sodium bicarbonate. Early in November, Papadogianis drew his blood and sent it off for analysis.

The results were devastating. John had harbored the hope that his body was free of cancer, especially after all the vitamin C treatments. But the German results showed that John had 31 million potentially cancerous cells circulating in his bloodstream, nearly half of which showed the markings of melanoma.

I have a copy of the report. It says the results show that John's body was rapidly making and unmaking cells, a sign that his immune system was working hard. It also says the melanoma cells that were in his bloodstream were likely from the original mole. The diagnosis: Melanoma. No therapy. Signed with best regards, Ulrich and Katharina Pachmann.

Together, John and Papadogianis started to plot out a whole new system of attack. Originally, they had thought a single series of vitamin C treatments might do the trick, along the same lines as a round of chemotherapy. Now, they began to think bigger. What if John needed to have infusions of vitamin C for a lot longer? They hit the intravenous bags hard again and kept sending blood samples to Germany.

The next test was better in some ways: only 8.5 million circulating tumor cells, but nearly 60 per cent were melanoma. Then John and Thea went to India and John was off the infusions for five weeks. He stopped in Frankfurt at the end of the five weeks to have a blood sample taken and sent to the Pachmann clinic in Bayreuth. The German technicians greeted him, "Yes, Mr. Patterson. We are expecting you."

By the time he got back to Papadogianis, the results were in and they were terrifying: 107 million circulating tumor cells. Papadogianis took another sample right away. Even worse. A steep rise to 131 million in a single week. The Pachmanns' analysis was stark. Increases of that magnitude could foretell a relapse — in John's case, the first metastatic tumor — in mere months.

The Chair, the Needle and the Bag

It was a cool Monday afternoon in October when I finally met Papadogianis. He wasn't scheduled to work that day but had come in because John wanted him to and because the two of them were committed to gathering data points in this experiment they were immersed in. Lanky, with dark hair and a quizzical smile, he moved fluidly around his treatment room carefully mixing up the bag of intravenous liquids, including 125 grams of vitamin C, imported from Galway, Ireland. John sat down in one of the brown leather chairs, joking that he's been there so often — two or three times a week — he figured he owns it.

Because I'm a Latin major, I'd come to think of Papadogianis as John's haruspex, that wonderful hybrid Latin and Sanskrit word meaning an ancient soothsayer, the one who can read the future. Haruspices were seminal members of a leader's court, the cherished, the privileged ones who had special knowledge, access and influence. They engendered faith. They are akin to today's top physicians at the world's best hospitals, like the surgeons who literally hold your heart in their hands and give you back life.

In Roman times, the leaders' questions usually had to do with a political rather than a medical future: who would win the battle or the war? And the highest manifestation of the haruspices' practice was the ability to read entrails. So the haruspex would slice open an animal — sometimes a human — and inspect its guts for a peek into the future. It was cutting-edge, important science for the day, right up there with the art of interpreting the mysterious words of oracles and reading the messages of the stars.

I'd been reading up on vitamin C and wanted to know why Papadogianis was such a believer. Since the early trauma after John had had what I came to think of as the "131 million scare," he had kept to a rigid schedule of treatments every few days with few interruptions, under

Papadogianis's strong encouragement. But Papadogianis struggled to point to a body of scientific evidence that supported vitamin C's benefits. So he talked about what he had seen in his own clinical practice.

Mostly, he said he used vitamin C on people who had advanced cancer and had already had chemotherapy. He said his observations led him to believe that the treatments made patients feel better for the time they had left, plugging into the hallowed and elusive quest to improve the quality of life of the dying. When pressed for examples, he mentioned one patient who had had surgery for stomach cancer and had terrible trouble eating or moving his bowels. He did some vitamin C treatments, changed his diet under Papadogianis's instructions and regained the ability to eat, gaining 10 kilograms.

Do the treatments extend life? I asked. He said, "Life expectancies and prognoses, I just don't go there." But he added, "I've never seen cancer cured."

All this time, John sat in his brown leather chair, hooked up to the intravenous bag. Papadogianis liked him to spend at least three hours with the drip and John was impatient with that. He kept cranking open the valve controlling the flow to make the fluids run faster. Two hours was about as long as he was willing to sit there. I pointed to the bag. What were its contents doing inside John's body right now? I asked Papadogianis.

The basic phenomenon is that the liquid vitamin C, also known as ascorbic acid or ascorbate, chemically reacts in the body to create hydrogen peroxide, he told me. Hydrogen peroxide is made up of two hydrogen atoms and two oxygen atoms. You can buy it as a cleaner for bathroom grout or for dousing cuts, but it's toxic if you put it straight into the body, either by mouth or vein. The interesting thing is that the hydrogen peroxide created in the body from intravenous vitamin C affects healthy cells and at least some cancerous cells differently. Healthy cells have an enzyme, called a catalase, that allows them to immediately discard or destroy the hydrogen peroxide, turning the two hydrogen and two oxygen atoms into harmless water and oxygen — $H_2O + O$. Cancer cells somehow can't do that. So the hydrogen peroxide kills some cancer cells while leaving healthy cells alone.

Papadogianis looked at me as though worried I wouldn't believe him, as if this would take a leap of faith, as I think it had for John. But the body of scientific literature on how intravenous vitamin C works has grown quite robust. A remaining puzzle is exactly why cancer cells react so catastrophically to hydrogen peroxide. Biochemists think it might have to do with the fact that the cancer cells, so perverted from their normal function, no longer have the protective catalyzing enzymes the healthy cells have and can't get rid of the hydrogen peroxide.

Possibly there are several oddities going on at the same time in cancer cells that combine to make hydrogen peroxide toxic to them, and it's probably different combinations in different types of cancer cells. Not all cancer cells respond, as a study by Melanie McConnell and others published in 2014 discovered. Worse, in some cancers, vitamin C will actually reverse the positive effects of chemotherapy when it's used at the same time, something no one wants.

But for whatever reason, the vitamin C seems to kill some cancer cells. A 2011 review paper and study by Mark Levine of the National Institutes of Health in Bethesda, Maryland, tried incubating normal cells and 43 types of cancer cells for an hour in a medium with differing concentrations of pure vitamin C. Healthy cells were unaffected. Three quarters of the cancer cell lines were partly killed off by the hydrogen peroxide when those concentrations got high enough.

When the same investigators tried infusing high doses of vitamin C into live mice implanted with human cancer cells of the ovary, brain and pancreas, they found that the vitamin C cut the tumors' size by half. Other animal studies — these are not clinical trials on humans — over several years have shown that tumors from colon cancer, sarcomas (soft tissues), leukemia (blood cancer), prostate cancer and mesothelioma (a type of lung cancer thought to be caused by asbestos exposure) have also shrunk with intravenous high-dose vitamin C therapy.

How high? A dose the equivalent of 1.5 grams of vitamin C per kilogram of human bodyweight delivered at a rate of half to one gram per minute. That led to a high concentration of vitamin C in the blood plasma for at least three hours, the Levine study shows. That's massively more than the 10 grams per treatment Pauling's 1970s studies used.

So far, studies on humans have shown few ill effects from even very high levels of vitamin C infusions, as long as patients with a history of kidney stones, kidney problems, anemia and the common enzyme deficiency known as G6PD (glucose 6 phosphate dehydrogenase deficiency) are not treated. However, a paper from 1979 reports that a patient treated with high doses of vitamin C died after the tumor collapsed rapidly and the site hemorrhaged. It seems to be a rare complication. The Levine paper said that based on surveys with naturopaths and other alternative doctors, and on sales of intravenous vitamin C, about 10,000 patients a year are treated in the U.S., with minimal side effects reported so far. But there's almost nothing in the medical literature that shows vitamin C on its own — without chemotherapy, too — has any effect on the lifespan of patients.

I noticed John was sleepy as the vitamin C flowed into him and almost incomprehensibly thirsty. He drank bottle after bottle of cold water from Papadogianis's fridge, darting up periodically to drag his intravenous pole with him to the bathroom. That thirst persisted for an hour or two after the treatment was done. But apart from that and fatigue and a vein in his arm that no longer wants to take an intravenous needle, he's shown few side effects.

THE TOXIC PRAYER

Vitamin C therapy brings to mind the history of those other chemical assaults on cancer cells, known as chemotherapy. The very idea that drugs could halt the growth of malignant tumors, or push back the advance of the few cancerous cells roaming the body, or cure cancer, was considered ludicrous by most people until the 1960s or 1970s. Until then, the treatments for cancer were surgery and maybe radiation. The field of medical oncology, which is the subspecialty of internal medicine devoted to using chemotherapy on cancer, did not even officially exist until 1973.

Yale University's Vincent DeVita, one of the giants of oncology and the former director of the U.S.'s National Cancer Institute, writes in the journal *Cancer Research* that in the 1960s, it took "plain old courage to be a chemotherapist." Some who tried to experiment with the drugs at that time were referred to openly as the "lunatic fringe." This was highly experimental, unpopular stuff. And like the remedies of the ancients — trying to readjust the humors by fiddling with the liquid elements of the body — it took a vibrant imagination.

You can see why it was frowned upon. The idea of chemotherapy came from the use of chemical weapons in war. DeVita reports that the original team of cancer drug researchers at New York's Sloan-Kettering moved there lock, stock and barrel from the U.S. government's Chemical Warfare Service after the Second World War. The first chemo drug was related to mustard gas. Doctors treating soldiers who had been gassed noticed that they died because their lymph nodes and bone marrow were terribly damaged. So early chemotherapists tried using derivatives of mustard gas in smaller amounts to kill off cancer cells in bone marrow as a way to treat cancer of the lymph system. The results seemed promising through the mid-1940s, but the remissions were "brief and incomplete," DeVita reports. But the early research led to a suite of similar drugs developed in the 1950s, some of which are still in use to treat some blood and lymph cancers.

By the early 1960s, researchers had begun looking to the plant world for treatments. One of the early successes was from the tiny Madagascar periwinkle, whose derivatives successfully treated leukemia (a blood cancer) and Hodgkin's lymphoma (a cancer of the lymph system). Since then, scientists have been scouring the world for plant remedies, including those used in traditional medicine. That's been dubbed "bioprospecting" or "biopiracy" and has led to criticism from indigenous peoples and farmers that heavily financed drug companies swoop in, find cures in the wild and make their billions without compensating those who found the natural drugs in the first place.

I remember being with an international cadre of bioprospecting scientists a decade ago, deep in the jungle of Suriname, once known as Dutch Guiana, in South America. They were on a collecting trip, following their hosts from the Trio tribe through the wilderness, trying to see in the plants what the healers of that ancient people saw.

One of the scientists on that trip told me of helping to find the breast cancer drug Taxol, which is derived from the yew tree. He remembered skinning tree after tree to get tiny amounts of the cancer-killing compounds they could distill from the bark to test the drug. When he and his team finally cracked the code of the yew's anti-cancer agent, he said they simply sat and stared at the beauty and complexity of a molecule they could never have imagined. He said that's why they plunder nature for medicine: evolution has developed compounds humans never could.

The problem with chemotherapy is that it doesn't discriminate between healthy and cancerous cells. It reacts the same way in both. So the concern has always been that it could do more harm than good. Even today, a small proportion of people die from side effects of chemotherapy. The drugs tend to attack the cells that are dividing rapidly, so that means the prolific cancer cells, but also healthy cells in bone marrow, the gastrointestinal tract, hair follicles and the immune system. That's why chemo patients are frequently bald, prone to infection and nauseated. Chemo is a medical gamble that enough healthy cells will remain to build those critical systems back up while the cancer scurries for cover. Sometimes it buys them time; sometimes it kills enough of the cancer to cure the disease.

Chemotherapy drugs were first used on people who were manifestly dying of cancer and for decades were the equivalent of a toxic prayer. But dosages and combinations have become far more refined over the past couple of decades and now chemo treatments can cure a handful of cancers and prolong the lives of those who have many types of cancer. The side effects are almost always severe. And while chemotherapy can sometimes work miracles, in other cases, it's ineffectual. It's also expensive. DeVita notes that it has turned into a multi-billion-dollar pharmaceutical industry.

By contrast, intravenous vitamin C seems like a relatively safe and inexpensive thing to test. Its cheapness is sometimes mentioned as a reason that it will never be tested in clinical trials: drug companies can never make enough money from it. But the financial winners, if it were ever to be shown to be effective, would be public health and medical insurance systems, which are in place in many parts of the world and which cover the heavy costs of chemotherapy. For example, a study published recently in the *Lancet Oncology* reported that the bloc of 27 European Union countries spends €51 billion a year on doctor services and drugs to treat cancer. Drug costs are a substantial part of treating cancer in Canada, too.

Not only that, but vitamin C also appears to be in the philosophical tradition of chemotherapy itself: promising, then derided, sometimes mocked and highly experimental.

The Levine paper, which was financially supported by the U.S. National Institutes of Health, comes to the conclusion that intravenous vitamin C is "ripe for investigation" as a drug for treating cancer, as long as it's in addition to traditional therapies such as chemotherapy rather than in place of them. The paper says that more tests on human subjects are the next logical phase of trial. And several small studies since 2008 on patients who had advanced pancreatic cancer (two of nine patients each and another, five) showed that intravenous vitamin C appeared to stabilize or diminish the tumors in some cases.

THE MEANING OF THE PATTERN

Papadogianis and John have made careful records of every treatment they've done. The only lapse in their data is that they have not measured John's blood plasma concentration of vitamin C after the infusions. On the October afternoon I was with him, John was getting 125 grams of vitamin C, which works out to about 1.1 grams for each kilogram of his weight. He was getting treatments every few days. But John and Papadogianis have experimented with lower and much higher doses and with frequencies. They shift it around according to how high or low the Pachmann count is, basing it on how his body appears to react rather than on an abstract dosage. A few times, they've done 300 grams (2.6 grams per kilogram of body weight) over the course of about seven hours but John felt unwell: his eyes stung, his mind was foggy. They abandoned it as a dosage.

Roughly every five weeks, they sent samples of John's blood to Germany and found an astonishing pattern. The more regular John's vitamin C infusions, the lower the circulating tumor cell count. When John slacked off the vitamin C infusions even for a week or two, or slid down to one treatment a week, the count went up, although it never again approached the fearsome 131 million reading. It was a lockstep equation and it didn't seem to be affected by fiddling with any of the other alternative medicines John was taking.

So what does that mean? The vitamin C trials in animals were on substantial tumors. John didn't have any tumors, so it was impossible to say that his had shrunk or changed in any way. His treatments were more experimental than any of the ones in the medical literature, or even in Papadogianis's practice. John's goal was to use the vitamin C to outwit the cancer, to make his body inhospitable to as many melanoma colonizers as possible. Did the rising number of circulating tumor cells mean more were on the move, searching for vital organs to invade? Did a lower number mean he had them on the run?

To John, it seemed reasonable that having more circulating tumor cells was bad and having fewer was good. In fact, that was the conclusion of the Pachmann lab itself, which said that a big increase meant, in essence, that a tumor could be forming. Nevertheless, John kept questioning what the counts really meant. Was this a reading of the entrails that had anything important to say about his future? Even though he was firmly committed to his twin therapies — vitamin C infusions and the Pachmann test — he kept coming back to me with the same question.

One of the conundrums: one of the times he had a

really massive intravenous vitamin C infusion of 300 grams over seven hours, he had his blood drawn right before and right after. Before, the sample showed he had 9 million circulating tumor cells including 6.3 million melanomas. After, it showed a huge spike: 34 million circulating tumor cells and 18 million melanoma cells. The Pachmann lab suggested that the big infusion of vitamin C had "flushed" the cancer cells into the bloodstream to be carried away.

None of it made any sense to me. Flushed from where? We were pretty sure John didn't have a tumor. He'd been having regular MRI (magnetic resonance imaging) scans, regular physical examinations to check for lumps. Nothing was showing up. The original mole site was healed and showing no signs of forming anything hard or suspicious. He'd had a long talk with his Toronto oncologist about the significance of the circulating tumor cell counts and how they fluctuated according to the vitamin C therapies. She found the trend interesting, but concluded, "At this point, there is no evidence available to show how the change of the number of these cancer cells would be correlated with the tumor."

I could understand the vitamin C. The science on that was gelling and the mechanism of how it works in the body was becoming clearer. Human tests were starting to emerge, even if they were mainly using the vitamin in combination with chemotherapy and were still inconclusive about big benefits. They were mainly finding that patients tolerated these megadoses of intravenous vitamins well, apart from the heavy toll they take on the kidneys. I worried that the duration and extent of John's treatments is so uncommon that the long-term effects on him are simply unknown.

But the counts of circulating tumor cells?

So I started to look into that, too. It was difficult for me. This was one of the two main planks of John's alternative therapy. He believed in both of them. Passionately. In fact, John and Papadogianis and their wives had even made a pilgrimage to Bayreuth, Germany, to see the lab and speak with Katharina Pachmann, and had invited her to Canada to give a lecture at one of the naturopathy schools, with a view to perhaps setting up a testing lab here. John believed in vitamin C because he felt he had proof of its effects from the Pachmann test. Thea told me flat out one night over dinner that John was still alive because he'd been taking vitamin C. And Papadogianis, John's haruspex, told me that their investigations so far led him to believe that John should keep up the vitamin C regimen forever. "We have control," he told me, sitting in his clinic in Barrie.

What if I found out something they didn't want to hear?

Chapter 5
Liquid Biopsy:
The Imagination of Cancer

Treating cancer has required imagination as well as knowledge as the centuries have passed. Consider breast cancer. In ancient eras, as in Egypt 5,000 years ago, it meant trying to envision how a tumor bulging out of the breast could be deadly. What was it doing to the rest of the body? What would cutting it out do? Or leaving it alone?

Much later, it took slicing away part of the tumor or sucking a bit of it into a biopsy needle and looking at it under the microscope, trying to understand what was going on inside those corrupt cells and how the new jobs they had created for themselves would affect the function of the whole body. Still later, it was trying to see tumors before you could feel them, taking x-ray pictures

— mammograms — of a breast to expose tiny, newly forming clusters of cancerous cells. And then, if necessary, surgically removing part of the breast, or all of it, and then treating the whole body with toxic chemicals — another leap of the imagination — to try to eliminate every last breast cancer cell hiding out anywhere.

Today, the divination has gone even further: finding the potential for cancer before the cell itself has figured out how to turn cancerous. Now, researchers can peer inside a woman's genetic code book to see whether she has a mutation that makes it likely she will get breast cancer in the future.

But what if the imagination could stretch just a little further? What if looking at what's in the blood could tell you whether you have cancer, and if you do, what the cancer's game plan is, how advanced it is or how it's reacting to treatment? It would be a snapshot that could be repeated literally hundreds of times if necessary, a moving picture to track what's going on at a cellular level, foretelling what will happen to the system as a whole. It's a radically different way of knowing about cancer than slicing a piece of tissue out of you at a single moment and looking at it, or trying to measure the size of a tumor through x-rays or magnetic images. Instead, this is a quest to read cancer's strategy within the transportation system it needs in order to spread to the vulnerable vital organs of your body.

That's the idea behind the Pachmann test and several dozen others developed over the past decade or so to scrutinize the composition of the blood and identify what are known as circulating tumor cells, markers of cancers that don't originate in the blood or lymph system. Dubbed the "liquid biopsy," the technique has been called one of the hottest new fields of cancer research, with more than 15,000 academic articles published by the middle of 2014 and hundreds more every year. The test holds out the possibility — not yet fully realized — of being able to diagnose cancer from a blood test.

The test might also be able to determine how cancer is reacting to treatment, and a lot of studies have looked at this already, focusing on breast cancer. Is a round of chemotherapy working? Instead of waiting weeks to measure the tumor, you could draw blood and see whether the circulating tumor cells were responding to treatment. Fewer meant treatment was working. The same or more meant it wasn't. Conceptually, at least. You could even find some of the tumor cells, snatch them from the cells around them, try to grow them in a lab and then try out different chemotherapies on them to see which ones work the best. That would represent a whole new era in cancer treatment.

The counts also hold out the possibility of tailoring dosages to the individual. Now, chemotherapy dosages are based on the maximum the body can tolerate without serious illness or death. But some cancers may be beaten back with a smaller dose, while others are immune to any amount. The circulating cells' reaction to treatment could determine how much is actually effective or whether no amount will be. The idea is promising enough that the U.S. government's Food and Drug Administration has approved one of the many emerging cell-counting methods for use in helping to assess treatments for metastatic breast, colorectal and prostate cancer: the Veridex CellSearch, owned by the personal care products company Johnson & Johnson.

The Philosopher's Stone

Even more tantalizing than blood biopsy or tracking the success of treatment — both of which can be done other ways, if not as easily — is the prospect that scientists could use the cells to predict what the cancer itself is going to do. This was John's hope. With the threat of a new tumor and no traditional medical treatment available to prevent one, he was trying to use blood counts to determine whether intravenous vitamin C was preventing his wandering cancer cells from taking root somewhere. He was trying to outwit the wily melanoma and, in some ways, the medical system itself, using emerging science to peer into the future of cancer treatment.

But do the counts really have the power to predict? I began to look at the evidence. I have to confess that the science on this — while fascinating — is so confusing and so unsettled that, as I write this, my brain is on fire trying to figure it out.

I've felt at times as though I had plunged into the midst

of an ancient race to find the philosopher's stone, the longed-for alchemical substance that would heal illness and prolong life, a quest peppered with proprietary secrets, bold dreams and would-be fortunes. Or perhaps into the pre-microchip era of the early 1960s when physicists were still trying to imagine a world with computers and couldn't solve the problem of the perpetually overheating room-sized machines. If only they could figure out how to cool computers down, the thinking went, the machines might really catch on. Eventually, of course, they made computer components smaller and then smaller still so that the need for cooling them down abated. The scientific dream, it seems, comes long before the perfection of technique.

The idea of cancer cells circulating in the body dates back to an Australian paper published in 1869 in which Thomas Ashworth reported noticing during an autopsy that he could find cancer cells in the bloodstream that were similar to the ones in the dead patient's tumor. He suggested that cancer used the blood to move around. The idea of finding cancer cells in the bloodstream has been hanging around the edges of cancer research since then, a tantalizing diagnostic dream.

The problem, then as now, is that there are so many white and red blood cells and very, very few circulating tumor cells. (Of course, this applies only to cancers that are not of the blood or lymph system, which can easily be seen in the blood.) A rough guess that runs through the medical literature is that there could be just a single circulating tumor cell for every 10 million white blood cells and 1 billion red blood cells. And the number of tumor cells is likely to vary from patient to patient and sometimes from time to time in a single patient, depending on the progress of the disease. David Parkinson and others have written a good review of the issues in a 2012 paper in *Journal of Translational Medicine*, and so have Bin Hong and Youli Zu in a 2013 paper in *Theranostics*.

Some studies have suggested that the number depends on how big the original tumor was and how recently it's been cut out. Cutting it out could release tumor cells into the blood, one theory goes. The number in the blood could also depend on how aggressively the cancer is replicating itself or how advanced the cancer is. There's no good information on how long those circulating tumor cells can live in the bloodstream — some reports say decades while others say hours — or how many a tumor might give off. So far, that's a big black hole. But the defining idea is that if there are any in the blood, the cancer has taken its first crucial step toward colonizing another part of the body by figuring out how to travel. If that's true, then it's a bad sign.

So the first challenge in trying to count cancer cells moving through the blood is to separate them from all those white and red blood cells. Getting rid of the red cells is straightforward and there's a standard protocol. But figuring out which of the remainder are cancerous and which are white blood cells (part of the immune system) turns out to be a fiendish and unsolved technological challenge to which many bright scientists are now applying themselves.

There's no standard way of even trying to do it. A recent paper listed 43 methods, none precisely the same, each bidding for commercial success. Some of the methods revolve around physically sorting cells according to characteristics like how big and how pliable they are. Cancer cells are often bigger than white blood cells and less pliable, but not always. Lots of these methods are being tested and they involve strategies like forcing them through tiny sieves or past different-sized pillars.

More common is to tag the cells with biochemical markers. The main way of doing that is to decide that the cancer cells in the blood are epithelial. Epithelial cells are the most common type of tissue cell in the body — the other three types of tissue cells are from muscles, nerves and connective bits — and they line body cavities and cover flat surfaces, including the skin. They're not too hard to identify because they have a molecular protein that not many other cells have and can be tagged, sometimes with magnetized beads or through other methods. Then they're sometimes labeled with fluorescent dyes for easier counting. Except some of the white blood cells they're surrounded with have the same protein. So the sorting then takes another turn: discarding white blood cells that look like epithelial cells by bonding them to another chemical marker that identifies them.

Recent studies, including those summarized in 2013 by Hongshen Ma and others in *Lab on a Chip*, a journal published by the Royal Society of Chemistry, are questioning whether this works all the time, but so far so good. The working definition of circulating tumor cells is epithelial cells that don't have the chemical marker for white blood cells.

The Strategy of the Cell

But are all the epithelial cells cancerous? The theory is that not very many normal epithelial cells end up in the bloodstream, so most of them must be cancer cells that have learned how to travel. Studies also show, though, that some of the circulating epithelial cells are healthy, not malignant. To make that plainer, the medical literature has taken to calling them "circulating epithelial cells," a nod to the fact that not all of them are cancer clones or from tumors at all. So that's one wrinkle in the counting system. It's not clear what's being counted.

Then there's the tricky business of whether the circulating epithelial cells that *are* part of the original tumor or a metastasized outlier are really poised to colonize. In order to make a thriving new metastatic tumor, the cells have to do more than break off from a tumor and cross into the bloodstream. They also have to be able to survive in the bloodstream, evading the body's immune system, and then figure out how to attach themselves somewhere else, how to clone like crazy and also how to build a blood system to feed the new growth. It's a pretty specific skill set. Which of the circulating epithelial cells are capable of doing all that?

That's another great puzzle. It's clear that some of them — maybe almost all of them — are gormless, just bopping around the bloodstream, with no intention of taking over other parts of the body. Finding out which ones have that colonialist intent takes not just crudely counting the cells, but looking even more closely inside them. Are they cancerous stem cells, for example, those self-perpetuating jacks of all trades that can make themselves into any type of cell that's wanted, anywhere? If one of those mutates into a cancerous version of itself, that's a problem because they have extra special powers of regeneration. And, according to some of the Pachmanns' work, cells have the ability to turn on and off their stem-cell-making capabilities. It's enough to make your brainpan melt.

Then there's the jarring recent finding described in the 2013 *Lab Chip* paper by Ma and others that the cells most aggressively poised to take the next steps on the road to metastasis no longer have the epithelial markers. They are flipping into a mesenchymal state, a state characteristic of connective tissue rather than epithelial tissue, and are therefore not caught by the net catching epithelial cells. The Ma paper called this a "fundamental flaw" in the current counting system.

So, not only is it not clear what's being counted, it's not clear what the cells that are being counted do, or that the right cells are being counted.

A Riddle Wrapped in an Enigma

When it comes to the Pachmann test that John has been doing, the complexities multiply. Both Katharina and Ulrich Pachmann, highly regarded German medical scientists, have written extensively in the medical literature about their methodology, called Maintrac, to which they hold patents. The patents mean that if their system gets picked up widely, they stand to make money. In the world of medical literature, that means they have a conflict of interest when they publish results describing their own method. They declare that conflict in their papers, according to publishing protocols, but because they stand to gain if their system wins out, it affects how people view their research. That's the first issue. The second is that their laser-scanning technique captures far, far more circulating epithelial cells than most other methods. In some cases, it's hundreds or thousands of times more.

Here's an example. The rule of thumb in much of the non-Pachmann testing world is that if a patient has more than five circulating tumor cells in 7.5 mL of blood, that's a dreadful sign of looming metastasis and death. John's very first Pachmann test, when he was so chuffed after the first run of intravenous vitamin C treatments and thought he might be cancer-free, found the equivalent of 47,625 circulating tumor cells in 7.5 mL of his blood.

Helpfully — or, terrifyingly — the Pachmanns translated that into a count of his body's estimated five litres of blood, which comes in at 31.75 million circulating tumor cells. And this is in John, who had an early stage of the disease. He had no distant metastasis. No new tumors. Other tests of circulating epithelial cells sometimes fail to find a single abnormal cell even in patients riddled with distant tumors.

The Pachmanns say in their writings that their way is simply more accurate, preserving the whole spectrum of potentially cancerous cells because they leave out one step that others do called "enrichment," which is meant to concentrate the cells of interest using such techniques as magnetized beads. But their method has been criticized in medical literature for overcounting. "Pachmann presents no proof that the observed epithelial cells are malignant tumor cells. Therefore it is possible that almost all of these cells are hematopoietic [blood-making] in origin," remarks Jonathan Uhr, in a 2004 letter to the editor critiquing the Pachmann methods in the journal *Clinical Cancer Research.*

While the Pachmanns say that they have substantiated their tests by running them on people who do not have cancer and finding no circulating epithelial cells, they have also found a substantial count in one person who doesn't have cancer: Thea. She and John were curious about the high counts in John, so they sent in a sample of her blood about a year after John began sending his. It found 3.75 million circulating tumor cells in her body, calling them "vital tumor cells," and saying that they are probably from a tumor, if she has a tumor, but that she needed to speak to a pathologist for a diagnosis. John said Papadogianis had encouraged them not to worry about the findings and they planned to have another test taken a few years later.

The Pachmanns, in turn, have criticized some of the other methods, particularly CellSearch, the sole approved method of counting in the U.S., saying they miss some critical cells. A few other studies, including the 2013 paper on trends in the research by Hong in *Theranostics*, say the same thing.

To make the whole field more confusing, the medical establishment, which could have endorsed the use of circulating epithelial cell counts and embraced the use of CellSearch, has largely held off so far on the grounds that it's not yet clear what the counts mean. Hong's 2013 paper lists the bodies that have rejected recommending it as part of diagnosis: the American Society of Clinical Oncology, the National Academy of Clinical Biochemistry and the American Association for Clinical Chemistry.

However, the heavyweight American Joint Committee on Cancer, which publishes the internationally recognized criteria for staging cancers and calculates the odds of dying with each stage (its system gave John the category of stage IIIb melanoma with a 60 per cent chance of being alive in five years), opted to incorporate the presence or absence of circulating tumor cells into its staging system during a review in 2010 (along with tumor cells detectable in bone marrow or randomly in other tissues). Here's the kicker, though: according to the new system, having circulating tumor cells doesn't change the stage of the cancer, meaning that at the moment, it's not clear what the significance is, if any.

The research is so perplexing, with 43 methods of counting circulating epithelial cells being developed for market as of 2012, that the Foundation for the National Institutes of Health Biomarkers Consortium in the U.S. has published a set of guidelines for every step of the process so that there will eventually be protocols to govern it. It's offering to coordinate the push for standards and clinical trials, saying the effort is too massive for any individual research institutions or private companies.

ON APPLES AND ORANGES

Into this mess landed the analysis from dozens of John's blood samples sent to the Pachmanns' German lab. And all this scientific chaos is only about how to count the epithelial cells in the blood, not about what the presence of those cells means, or about how the Pachmann lab sorts through the epithelial cells to find those that show up on John's reports as melanoma cells. Here's the third issue: the Pachmann lab has published many papers on its counting system but none on how it finds melanoma cells, meaning their methods haven't had the chance to be tested out by others. What are they looking for, exactly?

I finally asked Katharina Pachmann when she flew from Germany to Toronto to give a talk to some students, at John's behest and on his dime. It was an evening lecture and webinar at the Canadian College of Naturopathic Medicine, the dazzling new home of naturopathy in Canada. Papadogianis, who is one of Canada's leaders in complementing traditional oncology with naturopathic treatments, was there with John, me and a handful of others, totaling perhaps 15.

Pachmann, white hair caught in a flyaway bun, keen eyes flashing behind round glasses, explained to me afterward that her lab is checking for the melanoma A antigen in John's blood, but no other antigens. And she was categorical that her blood test cannot diagnose cancer but that she's convinced that most of the circulating epithelial cells she finds are cancerous, as long as the patient has already been diagnosed. In fact, her lab has figured out how to separate out individual cells and culture them in a soup containing that person's white blood cells to create what she calls "tumor spheres," a microtumor of cancer. The more cells capable of producing a sphere, the more advanced the cancer is, she's found. She's preparing a paper on this for publication.

But the medical literature makes clear that there are a handful of weird and devious molecular markers within the ribonucleic acid (RNA) of melanoma cells. They're unique to those cells but, of course, because it's cancer, not all the cells have all the markers all the time. They're hard to find.

Not only that, but there is no standard in the medical

literature for how to separate circulating melanoma cells from other circulating epithelial cells. In fact, a review study by Andrianos Nezos and others in *Cancer Treatment Reviews* in 2011 concluded that no single available technique and no single biological marker can sort out melanoma cells from any others. And a 2012 study by James Freeman and others in the *Journal of Translational Medicine* recommended that any test for circulating melanoma cells should screen for a whole bunch of markers if it's to be effective. In other words, while the Pachmann test may be overcounting circulating tumor cells, it could also be undercounting the ones that are melanoma.

But to the Pachmanns, who have published papers on how the circulating epithelial cells react to treatments for metastatic breast cancer, the information in the counts they're sending John is straightforward. They told Papadogianis that they have a research bank of findings from 13,000 patients telling them that a circulating epithelial cell count of 2 million or less in the whole body means the patient is not very likely to relapse or develop a new tumor; a count of 2 million to 10 million means the patient has a medium likelihood; more than 10 million means a relapse or tumor is imminent. Clear as could be. (Under this rubric, Thea has a medium chance of relapse from a cancer she doesn't have, by the way.)

I asked Katharina Pachmann about some of the things I was confused about. She was kind, almost merry. No tests are perfect when it comes to cancer, she told me.

Not CT scans, not MRIs, not pathology reports. And this is an emerging technology. But it's giving us information we didn't have before. Vital information that will help us manage the treatment of cancer over time, once we figure it out.

This may all fall in the realm of exciting medical discoveries, but to a lay researcher like me, it's devilishly confusing. I can see that eventually, if some of the technical issues get resolved, the investigation of circulating epithelial cells could transform our thinking about cancer, refine it, make us think about those traveling tumor bits differently. Perhaps the image will be of the immune system slapping the cells down like flies with a folded newspaper as they ineffectually try to replicate themselves, or monitoring them until their joyride in the bloodstream ends and they self-destruct. It's a profoundly different way of seeing cancer than the body lazily letting a single rapacious betrayer cell from within take over, different from the idea that even one rogue traveling cell is too many.

But the scene is not clear. Studies are pointing in different directions about what links there are between the circulating cells and the progress of the disease. It's so confusing that Liling Zhang and others published a meta-analysis of studies on breast cancer, in 2012 in the journal *Clinical Cancer Research*. It looked at 49 studies covering nearly 7,000 women, each of whom had at some point had blood taken and circulating epithelial cells examined. Most were counted using the CellSearch method, but other methods were allowed, too. It found that if circulating epithelial cells were present at all, whether the breast cancer was early or late stage, the patient did worse. However, the study could make no conclusions about the cell count's power to foretell the success of therapies. A flaw in the finding, Zhang and the other authors said, is that the detection of circulating epithelial cells is not standardized.

A paper the year earlier in *BMC Medicine* by Ramona Swaby and Massimo Cristofanilli that looked at several studies of women with advanced breast cancer whose blood was tested using only the CellSearch method concluded that lots of circulating epithelial cells — meaning more than five per 7.5 mL of blood — at any time during the disease was "an ominous prognostic indicator." Low levels of the cells meant that patients were more likely to survive or were responding to therapy. The paper concluded that for breast cancer, circulating epithelial cell counts were "a tool whose time has come of age."

Several studies of other types of cancer have shown a tendency for patients with a relatively high circulating epithelial cell count (more than three to five per 7.5 mL of blood) to succumb more quickly to cancers that had already metastasized. The problem for John is that none of these is comparable to the findings he is getting from Pachmann. It's apples to oranges.

The Anecdote Is Me

As I surrounded myself with piles of academic papers I'd marked up with colored pens, I realized that I'd been manically immersing myself in the math and the methodologies so I wouldn't have to think about John sitting day after day, week after week, month after month, in Papadogianis's brown leather chair, a needle in his arm, intravenous bag hanging on the pole above his head. I'd been avoiding thinking about how John and Thea felt, getting news from Germany every five weeks, avoiding thinking about how they reacted when they read those bare-bones charts translated from another language.

Sometimes it was a whipsaw. John frequently sent me text messages with the latest numbers, especially if they were triumphantly low. I know that his mood moved in tandem with the numbers. When they went up, he became reserved, maybe withdrawn. "It's the numbers," he would say. In some ways, those numbers from Germany shaped his life. It was as if the threat became more present for a few days, the dread crept up on him until he shook it off again.

I don't know how he kept going. All these papers, sorted by subject in untidy piles the length of my desk, cataloguing all these valiant, intelligent, creative efforts to treat cancer can't mask one fact: most of these patients have died from their rogue cell, despite the imagination, the tests, the treatments, the intensive scientific analysis. Their lives without disease are usually measured in handfuls of months, rarely in years.

Of all of them, the paper that hit me hardest is one published in November 2012 in the *Journal of Clinical Oncology* by Sojun Hoshimoto of the John Wayne Cancer Institute in Santa Monica, California, and others. That team was trying to find out if an experimental anti-melanoma vaccine would have any effect on the longevity of patients in precisely John's situation: stage III melanoma; metastasis in some sentinel lymph nodes; full lymph node removal; no medical treatment available; uncertain future. It turned out the vaccine didn't prolong life.

But as part of the long-running trial, they took blood from 320 patients after the lymph nodes came out and before they put them on the experimental treatments, and then tested the blood for circulating melanoma cells. They found them by probing deep into the mitochondrial RNA of the cells, the energy powerhouses that keep cells going, for several markers that only melanoma cells have. So they weren't looking for a count of cells, just a count of which markers, if any, the melanoma cells had.

Their finding is that patients whose cells carried more than one of the melanoma markers — only 10 per cent of the sample — were more apt to die early than those with just a single marker or none at all. But even so, nearly half of the patients with more than one marker were dead at five years and about a quarter of those with one or none. I know I should look at that and say that if we knew John were in the latter group, his chance of survival at five years would be 75 per cent or so, up from the 60 per cent he'd been given at the start. But the reality of writing about cancer is that sometimes the dark overcomes the light. And I know that if John is in the second group, his chances may be even lower than we thought. Usually, I can read the papers and say, But that's not John. John has a different stage, a different cancer. Not this time.

I want to be able to tell him he's on the right track, that he's going to be okay. But actually, I'm worried about how his blood tests are being done and what they mean. I know that he's had so many by this time that they can be compared to each other. He's actually got a bigger data set on his own cancer than any other I've seen in the published literature, both for vitamin C infusions and for circulating epithelial cell counts. It's a potential goldmine that might even have lessons for other patients, if anyone could figure out what they are.

But by now I'm so unconvinced by the methodology, and by the infant state of the field, that I'm not sure there's any significance in the test results he's been glued to. My faith, never a strong suit, is shot. It's possible that even without all his heroics, without the bags of vitamin C and all the other supplements he takes, John would be in precisely the same situation. It feels like a betrayal of both John and Thea even to admit this. So much for objectivity.

And it's impossible to know whether his regime is doing anything. In order to get any true sense of that, you'd have to have a whole group of people in precisely John's situation, give some of them intravenous vitamin C and others nothing and then watch them over time. Then you'd probably have to repeat it with a new group. Even then, there could be another factor that is influencing things more than vitamin C that we haven't thought of yet. Perhaps it's one of the other masses of alternative therapies he's taking, including mistletoe extracts. Maybe it's partly whether you believe that what you're doing makes a difference, or that you have some control over your fate, that it's not just up to the mythical sisters, spinning your life's length and then snipping it at a foreordained moment. And maybe it makes no difference what you believe.

Finally, I got both John and Papadogianis together in one room on Skype. John had just had a treatment and was woozy. Papadogianis was stubble-chinned and high-spirited, excited by the work he was doing with John, pumped by the potential that others could learn from his quest. I confessed my fears. What if John were to consult with some of the other blood testers, or the few people who are studying the clinical use of vitamin C? John and Papadogianis could hand over all their data for fresh analysis. Maybe these new specialists would have some more insight into John's future.

Papadogianis was sanguine. It would be 20 years before all my questions would be answered, he said. But before they had the Pachmann tests, the vitamin C treatments were just a roll of the dice. When they increased the frequency and fiddled with the dose, the counts came down. It had to mean something, even if we didn't know precisely what.

He said he approaches it emotionally. If he were to ignore the possibility of vitamin C's effectiveness, and the clues provided in the blood tests, and his patient got sicker, how would he forgive himself? I thought of the early chemotherapists who were trying so desperately to help their patients, believing that their experiments would lengthen their lives. Sometimes they did. Perhaps that's the nature of faith. Not that it's infallible, but that it determines a course of action for better reasons than anything else on offer.

John, looking impatient, leapt in. Where's the harm? he asked. He'd never had a day of illness or discomfort since he started taking vitamin C. True, he'd spent a whack of money — tens of thousands of dollars on these treatments alone so far — and been inconvenienced by all the time and energy it had taken. But did he want to experiment with cutting off the vitamin C and risk a tumor? No way.

But, I said, how do you know the vitamin C is making any difference or that the Pachmann tests are telling you anything significant? Where's the rigor of science?

John looked me straight in the eye, over thousands of miles of electronic impulses, from his iPad in Ontario to my laptop in Texas where I was on a fellowship to work on this book. "It's very personal and it's very anecdotal," he said. "But I happen to be the anecdote."

Chapter 6
Garden of Eden

Janus, Roman god of the gate, is two-headed, capable of looking both forward and backward at the same time. He is both sides of the coin, performing opposite actions simultaneously. Like his namesake month, January, he is responsible for beginnings, the magical moment when things can go either way. He is binary: both love and hate, triumph and defeat, birth as well as death. Above all, he is the god of possibility.

It strikes me that cancer is Janus-like. Diagnosis with cancer is the doorway into another life, an unsure one where the things you thought you could control are suddenly running amok. The certainty the post-war generations counted as a birthright — long, healthy living — is out the window, replaced by a crossing of the fingers. If you're lucky, things can go either way, forward toward health or backward toward further sickness. If you're unlucky, you move inexorably toward a death you never wanted. Cancer enhances your yearning for control while destroying the conviction you have any.

For John, that Janian duality played out in scale. While he was immersed in looking deep inside his secret blighted cells, in plotting tactics to forestall the actions of a single stealth colonizer that wanted to invade a new part of him, in relishing the cell-by-cell, day-by-day implosion of those miniscule melanoma clones circulating in his body, he was also putting in place a grand, decades-long scheme to turn his home county into a national leader in producing sustainable agriculture and energy.

It hadn't started out to be the bold public counterpoint to the private drama going on inside his body's molecules. In fact, it had started shortly before he was diagnosed with cancer the first time in late 2008, when the vision for what came to be known as Abbey Gardens was still just rumbling around in his head. He and Thea had returned to Canada after more than 30 years abroad, and had settled a three hours' drive north of Toronto in the county of Haliburton, a place famed for summer cottages, right on the boundary between the cultivated part of Canada and the wilds.

One of the things John noticed immediately was that very little food was grown locally, partly because the summers are shorter than in Ontario's more southerly primary agricultural lands and the winters longer. He would go to the supermarket, and the shelves would be full of fruits and vegetables from Chile or Mexico or California. He could practically smell their carbon footprint and pesticide residues in the atmosphere.

And as for energy, almost every bit of it was brought in from corporations or utilities. Hardly any was captured from the sun, the wind and the subterranean heat of the county itself. Garbage? It was something to get rid of, not something to turn into energy or use to grow food.

It was another way his life and mine had become linked. This is the area I've spent a lot of time researching and writing about for the past decade, and John and I routinely exchange information about the planet's stresses. In fact, one of the chapters of my first book stemmed from a tip from John: looking at Iceland's vow to rid itself of fossil fuels. And John had helped shape the final chapter of my second book by tutoring me on the nature of epiphany. I wrote a good chunk of that book one winter in Haliburton, holed up in a cabin he and Thea had built that was powered by the sun.

Like so many of us, he'd been anxiously tracking the environmental problems of the planet. It seemed like such an immense, unsolvable, uncontrollable problem. But it's been his gift to grasp possibilities others can't even imagine. So he started looking around, certain that groups of citizens could do something significant. I had told him about my visit to Eden, a garden named for the Biblical ground zero, built from a refurbished clay pit in Cornwall, the mythical land of Britain's Camelot. Eden was not only gardens, but also vast jungle-filled geodesic domes settled so deep in the pit that you come upon them unexpectedly as you draw near, oohing and aahing in pleasure. It has far-reaching education programs to teach citizens about where food really comes from and how to grow it. John made a trip to Eden and came back with visions of domes and organic tomatoes dancing in his head.

Shortly after that, he happened upon a gravel pit, nearly exhausted, on an 85-hectare (210 acre) patch of land just a few kilometers down the road from his home in Haliburton County. To others, it was high piles of small stones scraped out of scourged earth, shortly to be made into highways. To John, it was the cradle of inspiration and beauty, a place where the whole community could pull together to tackle the excesses of civilization and show the world how it could be done.

It started taking off as his melanoma was diagnosed, just at the start of his critical five-year dash to keep himself alive. The two dreams — both of which he talked about openly — seemed to feed each other: killing off the cancer and nurturing the abundance of his Eden. Death and birth in the same breath.

That first melanoma year was the year of the first small market garden. It grew enough organic vegetables and herbs to feed a farmer's market that a delighted John had also helped bring to life. No longer did we take him organic vegetables to stave off the cancer; now, he sent them home with us.

That was the year the first whack of money came in from the local development agency, earmarked for a study to see if John's wild idea could get off the ground. And John said, Why not organic meat to go with the vegetables? So Abbey Gardens began raising fat chickens — reared for the delicate first few days in John's garage — then fatter turkeys.

And then the local college sent in a team to build a community kitchen and food hub out of straw bales, heated and cooled with energy from below the Earth's crust, a gathering place where citizens could sell food they grew, buy it or learn how to cook it. All of a sudden, others in the community were growing their own food, taking some of it to markets, dreaming about a world in which their neighbors farmed energy, too, fed it to the power grid and kept carbon out of the air. It was a place where waste was no longer wasted, but turned into something people needed. It was as though they longed for a world where they could push back the forces that were spinning it toward chaos and that Abbey Gardens could become its epicenter.

I think I underestimated how much the metaphors of cancer and environmental destruction had become merged — probably subconsciously — for all of us who were pulling for John's garden. And maybe it went much further than that. As Mukherjee says:

"Every era casts illness in its own image. Society, like the ultimate psychosomatic patient, matches its medical afflictions to its psychological crises; when a disease touches such a visceral chord, it is often because that chord is already resonating."

Mukherjee traces the roots of modern society's psychological crisis to a shift in the early 1970s from an external horror, such as the Cold War, to an undefined internal horror — he points to a vague spiritual decay — that threatened both society and individuals.

In other words, society has a pattern of creating meaning for why disease happens, unconnected with the physical causes of the disease. In this case, it is cancer, the disease we understand so poorly. But while the psychic horror that makes the chord resonate might once have been vague, I don't think it is anymore. I think the psychological trauma stems from the increasing scientific understanding of how our species has affected the life-support systems of the planet.

There's a scientific drumbeat telling us, in so many words, that our species is a cancer, killing the world as we know it, fouling waters, felling forests, changing the chemistry of the atmosphere and the ocean, destabilizing things. And the time frame for destruction grows ever nearer as scientific predictions for disaster are shown to be too conservative. Once, Armageddon was pegged to occur about the end of this century. Now, it's within mere decades. Not our grandchildren, but us.

And it's no longer merely conceptual. We can see the

effects of the destabilization with our own senses: the east coast's Superstorm Sandy, tsunami-like deluges in Alberta, California's drought, the west coast's oyster and scallop fisheries destroyed by acidic seas.

When it came to Abbey Gardens, the merged cancer/environment metaphor became intertwined with the metaphor of the garden, the unspoiled, life-giving place where needs are met, where everything is in order, destined to last as long as we take care of it.

Cancer and environmental distress on one side, the garden on the other. It was Janus again, both the loss of control and the attempt to regain it.

LUMP IN THE NECK

My daughter, Calista Michel, who was finishing her first degree in English literature, was drawn to the garden. John invited her to Haliburton to work there the summer after he was diagnosed with melanoma, and again the summer after that. She borrowed my car each summer and drove three hours north through Toronto's ferocious traffic and then onto the back roads, through farms and forests. Every single time, I was paralyzed with visions of a traffic accident that would see her injured or dead. Every time she arrived, I would breathe a sigh of relief. The terrors of watching a first child become independent.

Husbanding the chickens became a big part of her work, and Calista, home every few weekends to visit, would regale us with tales of the birds' escapades. One evening, she and John arrived to usher the birds back into the coop for the night, only to find that they had figured out how to rootle around under their fence and escape into the garden next door. There they were, munching away on organic beet greens and lettuce, having their fill of the plants the garden team had coaxed so painstakingly to market size. John held up the fence and Calista chased the chickens back to their own side and then into the coop.

Near the end of her second summer, she and I were making dinner at home and she was laughing uproariously, chin raised in the air. I noticed a lump on her neck. You might be brewing a cold, I told her. Better push the fluids. But when she finished the summer job and returned home for the school year, the lump was still there. Do me a favor and get that checked out, I said to her.

She was good-natured about it and went off to the doctor, who wasn't very worried but sent her for an ultrasound and some blood tests. The ultrasound showed a node in her thyroid and within a week, she and I were at the hospital for her appointment with an endocrinologist.

She was 21 and I thought it was pretty generous of her to let me go with her. I stayed in the waiting room and told her if she needed me, to send someone out. I'd done a skiff of research and had found that nodes in the thyroid are common. I wasn't on high alert. In fact, I dozed off for a moment while I waited, reading a magazine. And then something changed. I can't say what it was, but all of a sudden I was tense and vigilant, eyes pinned to the door. A moment later, a tall doctor rushed into the waiting room, calling for Calista's mom. Without a word, I followed her, racing down the hall.

Calista, usually so composed, was sobbing, hysterical. I cradled her in my arms. The second doctor held a needle. She'd just finished taking the third exquisitely painful biopsy out of the hard node and she looked grim. She'd already summoned a technician to come to the room and hand-deliver the biopsy samples to the hospital's pathology department for a rush analysis and the technician burst into the room, took the package and raced out. It's a massive tumor and we think it's cancer, the second doctor told me. And if it is, that thyroid will have to come out next week.

I don't know how we stumbled home. I remember clutching Calista by the waist, trying to weld her to me as we walked to the subway, saying over and over again that maybe it wasn't cancer and even if it was, we wouldn't let it define her life. We limped through the next few days until the phone call came.

All clear. The biopsies were negative. Calista would only need to have half her thyroid out — the tumor was so big it was pressing on her windpipe and vocal chords — and that could wait a few weeks until her school schedule was more flexible.

I hadn't collapsed until then. But I cried as I have rarely cried in my life. Deep, gulping sobs of relief. Now all we had to do was get through the surgery: tricky, because it was so near the vocal chords, spinal nerves, the carotid artery and the jugular vein; long, because the tumor was so large. But so, so much better than surgery for cancer.

There were families of other patients in the waiting room during the long day of Calista's surgery — people whose loved ones were lying on operating tables just meters away with teams of medical people hanging over them, cutting cancerous tumors and flesh out of their bodies.

I remember one young man whose wife was having a mastectomy that day, thinking, so, so selfishly, that I was glad it wasn't me spending all those hours envisioning the surgery of my loved one, wondering if the surgeon had captured enough clones of the rogue cell. Wondering if my beloved would live.

He seemed so calm about her, resigned. I could pick up no energy from him at all, except that he was obsessed with charging up his cell phone and laptop computer. He was working away on a file, making phone calls to clients, like it was just another day at the office. I was reading a mystery novel, desperate to keep the images of what was happening to my daughter out of my head.

It was weeks later, after the deep red slash across her neck had begun to heal, that Calista and I ended up at the hospital again for a routine chat with the surgeon who had taken out half the thyroid. She walked in the room with the chart, read it carefully, squared her shoulders slightly, looked me fiercely in the eye, then turned to Calista. The biopsies were wrong. This is cancer. You have to have another operation to take out the other half of your thyroid and maybe some lymph nodes. And then you'll be treated with radioactive iodine to try to eradicate every last thyroid cell in your body.

TRAPPED IN THE METAPHOR

Something in you dies when you find out your child has cancer. It is not a subtle death. It is noisy and wet and rancorous. I had a long-planned dinner party set for a couple of days after we got the diagnosis, and realized I couldn't go through with it. I phoned my friend to cancel and found myself unable to talk, overcome with a pain I had never experienced before. Finally, I got the words out. A moment later, I was curled up on the floor keening. I have no other way to describe it, those wails of anguish surging from me in a voice I didn't recognize.

Above all, I felt guilt. That it ought to have been me instead of my first-born. That I ought to have been able to forestall this somehow. That I hadn't fed her enough organic greens or kept her away from enough radiation. Obsessively, I replayed every second of her childhood that I could remember, wondering what I had done to fail her in this way.

My belief in the value of lucid scientific inquiry, of careful data points was blasted away. All the detached analysis I thought I had gained during my two years as John's cancer broker, my clear-eyed parsings of the data, my excavations of the myths that society constructs around cancer — gone.

My self-righteousness that I was getting to the root of this metaphor that has society in its thrall, identifying how it's subverting our energies in ways we barely identify — vanished. I was trapped in what Sontag calls the lurid metaphors that inhabit the landscape of the kingdom of the ill — the guilt-embroidered fantasy.

It didn't matter that I could see the metaphor, follow its veins through the flesh of society. I was in its grip.

The urge to take on the blame was overwhelming. It was critically important to me that this not be random, that it not be just a cell that had decided on a whim to rewrite its instruction manual. All this pain had to have a higher meaning. It was somehow a punishment for my secret failings.

Looking back now, I think it was a way of trying to regain psychological control. This cancer seemed to have so much more meaning than, say, a broken arm or a bout of pneumonia, both of which I had dealt with before as a parent. Those were worried and watchful times, but not freighted with guilt like this. If I couldn't point to a clear reason it had happened — not soot or tobacco or asbestos, for example — I wanted to be able to point to something in me. Not knowing why it had happened was so much scarier than being able to say that I had done something wrong. If there were no reason, I would never be able to let the fear go. It would haunt me forever, a ghost I could never lay to rest.

Calista didn't feel guilt. I guess being 21 was her free pass. Plus, the doctors had told us about the global uptick in thyroid cancers, particularly among young women, for reasons no one had uncovered. She felt shame when several well-meaning university friends told her she had cancer because she had not spoken up enough in her life. Her throat was literally closing up as punishment for repressed thoughts, unsaid emotions, they said.

That hit home because it plugged into our family lore, not exaggerated, that her grade-school teachers never heard her voice until the final week of classes. And she certainly was the recipient of pity and prejudice. Her boyfriend refused to visit her at the hospital after the operation and categorically rejected helping her through the radioactive period. She dumped him. We opened champagne.

Just to explain how out of proportion my reaction was, let me note that Calista's cancer was one of the few that, as far as the doctors were concerned, was as close to curable as any cancer ever gets. In a panic, I called my brother Ross Mitchell, a medical biophysicist at the Mayo Clinic in Arizona, and his wife, Sheela Hota-Mitchell, a microbiologist. After some research, they told me their oncologist buddies at the Mayo never even saw thyroid cancer patients. It was all dealt with by regular non-cancer surgeons because it so rarely got to be a life-threatening problem.

Not only that, by the time we found out that she had cancer, the tumor was no longer in her body. A week after the diagnosis from the surgeon, we went back to see the two endocrinologists again and all that became clear. I still have my pencil-written notes from the meeting — it lasted more than an hour — with our list of questions and their answers.

This was a stage I papillary thyroid cancer. It hadn't spread to the lymph nodes or anywhere else. It was still contained within the gland in its own capsule, according to Calista's pathology report describing the large piece of her that had been sliced out and preserved in formalin. All good news. The cancerous cells had a weird architecture, called macrofollicular, which was why the biopsies hadn't caught it. But that architecture was also characteristic of the least aggressive form of thyroid cancer. This was not a careerist, inventive, travel-prone cell. It was, at this point, rather sedate and content with its lot in life. But given enough time, that kind of cancer could dream of an empire.

I wanted to know how long it could have hidden in there before it metastasized. The doctors couldn't say. We didn't even know how long it had been there. We actually went back to old photographs to see if we could find evidence of it in her neck in earlier years. Nothing obvious.

When it came to the threat to Calista's life, the doctors were categorical: there wasn't one because she was so young and because they'd caught it early enough. She would live. She would not die of this cancer.

The numbers on the thyroid cancer calculators of the American Thyroid Association and the American Cancer Society show that the critical thing in Calista's type of cancer is the age at which it's diagnosed. Before 45 and it's pretty much curable, even if it has spread, which hers had not. According to the math, Calista's survival rate at five years is 100 per cent and at 20 years is at least 99 per cent.

They are very good odds. And I know that my scientific brain believes them, if not my panic-ridden, maternal one. Those odds should have made a difference to my reaction. I should have been able to take the diagnosis calmly, intelligently, reflectively. But that would be to assign rationality to this phenomenon. The trouble with abject fear — with searing, lurid metaphor — is that it is not rational. And the myths that spring out of fear that deep are certainly not. They are the stuff of nightmares. They are tenacious.

Soundless and White

Calista and I had been through a medical crisis before, just as she was being born, which is perhaps why this one echoed so strongly. The last day she was inside me, I felt that something was wrong. I was on watch, home from work, cervix partially dilated, waiting for my waters to break. But I couldn't feel her move that last morning. I had been an inveterate kick-counter, fearful that I would lose her ever since an unexplained hemorrhage early in the pregnancy. I felt I had made a psychic deal with this baby growing inside me: I will listen and count and you will stay alive. And then this day, just as I hoped she was getting ready to be born, no movement.

My obstetrician was reassuring and suggested I meet him at the hospital for an ultrasound. It was the end of July and I remember the oppressive wet heat, the voluminous red dress I was wearing, swollen feet squashed into red shoes that would normally have been too big for me. I called a taxi and sat on the front steps to wait for it. The baby moved spasmodically several times — jerks — the minimum requisite number. Those were the days before cell phones and I was too pregnant to go back upstairs and cancel the taxi. And things still felt strange. So I waited.

By the time I got to the hospital, the ultrasound clinic was closed for lunch. I waited again. Finally, the technician smeared lubricating gel over my belly and began to peer inside my uterus with sound waves. The baby was not moving except for a sinusoidal heart rate. A sign of acute distress. I remember the technician slapping my belly, trying to make enough noise to prod the baby into moving. Nothing. Things became silent and efficient and swift after that. They plopped me into a wheelchair and took me a few floors up to the delivery room. My obstetrician was pacing in front of the elevator doors. "Alanna," he said, grasping my hands, looking me intently in the eye. "We have to do a caesarian section. Right now." I told him I understood, but that I needed to go to the bathroom first. "Oh, Alanna," he said. "We have no time for that."

Maybe not even enough time to give me an epidural anesthetic, they said. Every second counted. And then they decided they would try, but only once. And if it didn't take, they would slice into me without anesthetic. I didn't care. My eyes were glued to the heart-monitor they'd strapped around my belly, praying to every god I'd ever read about or imagined that the heart would keep going until they cut her out of me.

She was unearthly white when she finally emerged, muscles eerily uncoiled, overstretched heart unmoving. Soundless.

Hours later, long after they got her heart moving again, the story began to emerge. My placenta and umbilical chord were horribly malformed and had allowed her to bleed nearly all her blood into me over months, probably. She survived with less and less blood and less and less oxygen as the months went on, her tiny heart enlarging dangerously as it tried to get what little blood there was to where it was needed. My organs that were supposed to keep her alive were also slowly killing her. Janus.

Another hour, my doctor said. Just one more hour and she would have been dead.

The cold terror of it strikes me even now: if I'd slept in that morning; if I'd forgotten to count; if I'd waited to call the obstetrician; if he hadn't taken me seriously; if I hadn't; if I'd canceled the taxi; if the ultrasound clinic had been busier; if the operating rooms had been full; if I hadn't happened to live in a big metropolis with a neonatal intensive care unit at the ready.

Throughout those long days afterward, as they transfused her and checked to see whether she had any brain damage and pumped her with antibiotics to combat an infection she'd gotten after birth because her immune system was shot, the nurses trooped through my hospital room to see the mother who had had a miracle birth.

Once I knew she would survive, the hell of not knowing why it had happened descended on me. I reran every moment of the pregnancy — stop, replay, stop, replay — trying to figure out what I had done wrong. The doctors questioned me closely about my pregnant life. In the end, they decided it was just something random. No reason. No blame. No penance. Worst of all, no redemption.

I could never accept it. Even now, writing about it for the first time in this detail, I've been checking through the latest medical literature on extreme newborn anemia, looking at the unutterably shocking statistics on how many babies die who have what Calista had — almost every single one — and how many others are profoundly neurologically damaged if they live — most.

I know that when I tacked all my courage to the wall and decided to have a second child, the obstetrician who handled the case twice looked up during the initial appointment from the medical notes on Calista's birth to ask me if she had survived. Twice I said she had.

He couldn't believe it. He was head of the hospital's high-risk obstetrical section and he had never heard of a baby who had bounced back from that sort of blood loss.

For the next 21 years, I agonized about protecting her from any further harm. I figured she'd already been through more than her share. But, as it turned out, I couldn't protect her from cancer, our modern plague. Now this child who had had to be cut out of me to dodge death had had to have something cut out of her in order to save her life again. Janus.

For the first time, I understood the ancients' need to find explanations for why things happen. It's a quintessential human imperative. Random is not emotionally satisfying. Therefore, lightning was the bolt from an angry god. Crop failure was punishment for failing to honor the gods with a fatted calf. The plague happened because you took the Lord's name in vain or coveted your neighbor's wife. Going to church regularly and praying could forestall illness. And on and on.

The point is that if you think you can pinpoint the cause, then you can fool yourself into thinking you can avert the cause. It's deeply egotistical. It's life played as a grand insurance policy. Our myth-making around cancer stems from the same impulse. Because we don't know exactly why most of it happens, we weave a makeshift wisdom around it, a false prophet, which seeps into the common story and feeds our hunger to understand why. The guilt is a byproduct, a way to assign blame and seek absolution. It's a lesser evil than the forces of randomness. And it gives us the illusion of control.

Eventually, I pulled up. I looked again and again at the statistics and took tentative steps toward having faith in them and in the system that had produced them, the one I had believed in all my life. Calista's endocrinologists were anxious that she have radioactive iodine ablation therapy, meaning getting rid of all her thyroid cells whether they were cancerous or not.

It was another act of faith. Eating even extremely low doses of radioactivity — in her case 30 millicuries, named after the Nobel Prize–winner Marie Curie who discovered radium and died from exposure to it — carries modest risks of causing cancer in salivary glands, breasts and the bladder. But while getting thyroid cancer so young meant it wasn't as dangerous as getting it when she was older, it also meant Calista had more decades for the cancer to return. Her doctors wanted to wipe the thyroid slate as clean as possible and monitor her rigorously for the rest of her life, so they could tell if any thyroid cells were growing back.

It happens that thyroid cells are some of the few in the body to absorb iodine. So you can target them. The theory is that if you take out as much of the thyroid tissue as you can surgically, then artificially make the cells thirsty for iodine and then introduce radioactive iodine into the body, any hidden, scattered thyroid cells will suck the iodine in and be executed by the radioactivity. It's a similar principle to intravenous vitamin C therapy, except the target isn't all cancer cells, it's all thyroid cells. So Calista went on a rigid low-iodine diet for a few weeks — no salt, nothing from the sea, no dairy, no soy — and then showed up at the hospital again.

This time, they shut her in a lead-lined room by herself, handed her a lead cylinder coated in yellow — the universal color for radioactivity — and told her to swallow the pill it contained. She was dangerous to others for a week, literally untouchable, cloistered in a room, needing separate dishes and bathroom, and banned from using electronics lest she foul them with her touch.

A follow-up scan and blood tests to check for the presence of thyroid hormones didn't show quite the eradication her doctors were hoping for. So, nearly a year later, she went into the same lead-lined room and had another dose — just 4 millicuries this time — so they could do another in-depth scan, searching for hot clumps of thyroid tissue.

This time, all was well.

Nearly two years after I noticed the lump in her neck, we went back to the endocrinologists and they told her they liked her numbers. No further surgery. No more radiation for now. Lifelong monitoring. But cancer-free.

My throat closed up with emotion so strong I couldn't speak for half an hour.

Chapter 7

Rewriting the Metaphor

Metaphors are sneaky. They infuse the way we think about things without our noticing. And then they start to define reality. And then that influences how we act. And much of it, under the radar, subconscious. Reinforcing itself. A self-fulfilling prophecy.

I was struggling with the whole concept of what metaphor really is and how it works, so I went back to *Metaphors We Live By,* by George Lakoff and Mark Johnson, a classic piece of scholarship first published in 1980. They start the book with an example that has become a linguistic standard: unraveling the metaphor embedded in the idea that argument is war.

What they mean is that the language we use to describe arguing is the same as the language we use to describe war. Arguing is war. So we attack weak points in arguments. We demolish an argument. We use strategies as we argue. We shoot down arguments. We defend our points. We gain ground or lose it. We have lines of attack. We win and lose arguments.

So far so good.

But then, to illustrate the idea further, Lakoff and Johnson ask us to imagine a society where the cultural understanding of argument is dance instead of war. So when people argue, they're not concerned about who wins or loses. They're performers. They are immersed in giving a balanced, gracious, emotionally fulfilling performance.

An argument based on the metaphor of dance would feel different from the arguments we experience in our less noble moments as we do battle with, say, a driver who steals our parking spot. Or the disputes we see captured on film and television, whose participants are frequently "explosively" angry and, if they lose, are "sore" about it and "nurse their wounds."

The larger point is that an argument founded on the metaphor of dance would not just feel different, it would also be different. Metaphor is not just about words. It is also about thought processes and actions. It is about reality.

In the case of cancer, the metaphors are layered. They govern how we think about what cancer is, how prevalent we think it is, how much control we think we have over getting it and living with it, whether we feel responsible for having it.

The predominant cancer metaphor is war. We fight cancer, usually valiantly. We attack tumors and try to annihilate them and bring out our arsenals to do that, and so on. It's us against cancer. This metaphor has come in for its share of criticism within the ethical, psychological and even oncological disciplines. A main concern is that when someone dies of cancer, the message that remains is that that person just hasn't fought hard enough, was not a brave enough soldier against the ultimate foe, did not really want to win.

The cancer-is-war metaphor does not seem to allow space for the idea that in actual war, some soldiers die heroically for the larger good, no matter which side wins. War is death. In the cancer war, if you die, you've lost and cancer has won. The dead are responsible not just for getting cancer, but also for failing to defeat it.

Of course, many cancer patients who die would much, much rather have won. That means some cancer professionals and patients balk at the war metaphor, feeling it does patients and their loved ones a disservice, that it impugns them unfairly, that it does not acknowledge the limitations of cancer research and treatment and even our understanding of how cancer works. "I want my patients to be fighters," said an oncologist during a discussion by health-care providers at the Massachusetts General

Hospital published in the *Oncologist* in 2004. "But, I want them to fight for the right thing. You can fight for courage, loyalty and living well. . . . The question is at what point are you still holding on to your metaphor in the wrong fight."

Not all cancers can be beaten, as it stands now. This is frequently a fatal disease no matter how militaristic the attempts to defeat it, no matter how hard the fundraisers try to spin the nearness of total cure.

A research paper by David Hauser and others published in 2014 found that the war metaphor can actually impair some people's enthusiasm for avoiding cancer risks. People who are fighting wars, he points out, are not in the mindset of holding back and carefully assessing their actions or, in cancer-speak, eating more organic broccoli and losing 10 pounds.

But the cancer metaphor is both richer and more nuanced than that. A war is something that one gets swept up in. It is a large social endeavor. Everybody is affected some way, pulling for a win by, say, planting victory gardens and knitting woolly caps. That's the metaphor the money-raising arms of cancer plug into, right from the U.S.'s first National Cancer Act, signed into law by then-president Richard Nixon in 1971. As Richard Penson and others write in a 2004 paper, the language was explicitly militaristic, a piece of legislation that "mobilized the country's resources to make the conquest of cancer a national crusade." The whole society was fighting the ultimate foe, which was cancer.

But also embedded in the opulent metaphor of cancer is an opposing idea: if you get cancer, it's your fault. So it's not really a society-wide endeavor at all. It's a private war within your body that you're to blame for, one that costs society billions in what the economists call the financial "burden" of cancer. You're screwing things up for everybody, costing us all money, stripping our economy of your productivity, seeding fear that others will get what you've got. If only you'd been able to control yourself — eaten more organic broccoli, say, and lost those 10 pounds — we wouldn't be in this mess. It's Janus, the Roman god of the gate, all over again. Two opposing things happening simultaneously.

Of course, there's more. According to one powerful guilt-inducing line of reasoning, if we don't personally donate more money to find cancer cures, we're letting everyone down, too. Take the Stand Up to Cancer (SU2C) campaign, the one that enlists the cream of Hollywood to deliver its messages, the one trying to raise yet more money for cancer research. It has cannily plugged into the fear and dread that so many of us feel, all the while averring that cancer cures are just around the corner if only we would step up to the plate: "Cancer takes one person every minute. . . . Every day in America 1,500 people die despite the fact that the means to save them are literally within our reach. To wait any longer for someone else to save our lives and the lives of those we love is unforgivable. We must act now." A manifesto on the site, written in the form of a poem says: "We are a tapestry of lives touched and brought together by a terrorist we can actually find."

According to this line of reasoning, every time anyone dies of cancer it's because we, as a society, haven't fought hard enough. Our actions in letting someone die of cancer, it says, are unforgivable. We've failed to mobilize our arsenal against, not just the ultimate foe, but the terrorist, the one that would bring down our cherished way of life. But — here's Janus again — cancer is also cast as the disease of our civilization, the one we've created by our communal actions, the one that is endangering us all. This thinking is fed by the environmental crisis our planet actually is in, which scientists tell us our species has spawned. Humans are literally akin to a cancer on the planet's life support systems, pushing its life forms toward a spasm of extinction by our actions and refusing to make things better.

It's helpful to me to unpack these ideas by comparing the ways our society sees cancer with how we position heart disease and stroke, the other big killers. It's hard to imagine seeing, say, stroke as the ultimate enemy of civilization, the "terrorist" that is poised to get us all, that has all of us in the grip of dread. The closest we've come is to try to pin the blame on salty fast foods as a trigger for high blood pressure and to lobby manufacturers to use less salt. It doesn't amount to the same sickening disquiet.

These cancer metaphors — and, of course, there are more of them — overlap and contradict each other, ping-ponging back and forth, a sign that we are struggling to explain something we don't fully understand. That's why we can hold the three impossible beliefs about cancer all at the same time: inevitable, preventable, deserved.

Does this grim servitude to the cancer metaphor matter?

It's hard to know precisely, hard to calculate its effects. Exactly how does it hold us back? I've come to believe that the cancer metaphor makes many of us feel more vulnerable than we are, less in control than we actually are. It's like the sword of Damocles suspended over our heads. One wrong move and, bam, done. There's the sense that we are under the control of an invisible tyrant poised to pounce; we must dutifully follow the dictates of a bewildering, shifting anti-cancer screed or else we have failed not only ourselves, but also our society.

I think the brutality of the cancer metaphor saps our society of some of its productive vigor. Guilt and blame and fear are paralytic emotions, a black hole for energy. Certainly the prevailing view of cancer adds unnecessary pain to the lives of those who are already struggling with serious disease, whether in themselves or in a loved one. I think it sows anxiety in our society, plugging into our fears about whether we've created a civilization that can last, or whether we've made something toxic, death-dealing.

I find evidence for that in the studies reporting widespread stigma among cancer patients. People who liken having cancer to having leprosy in the Middle Ages. People whose friends refuse to visit or cross to the other side of the street when they catch sight of them. It's in those doctors and nurses in the British study who drew their cancer and AIDS patients as faceless, dehumanized figures with their vital organs spilling out of incomplete outlines, their very selfhood erased. It's in the fact that even though we know so much more today about how cancer works and about how to lengthen the lives of those who have it, as a society, we fear it at least as much as we did nearly 40 years ago when Sontag wrote *Illness as Metaphor* and pleaded for liberation from the disease metaphor.

We have inflated ideas about how much cancer there is and how much risk we're at right now, some of which are exploited by people who want to raise money for "the cure." Walk up to nearly anyone on the street and ask about cancer and you'll hear that it's far more prevalent today than it ever was. But there's more cancer because cancer is a disease of the elderly and we have more elderly in the world. And we have more people. If you adjust for age and the growth in the population, there's less cancer than there was even a few years ago in the Western world — with some exceptions like lung cancer in women and thyroid cancer — and it tends to be less deadly. You could argue that cancer is on the wane, on the run.

I hear the cruelty of the cancer metaphor in the fear-filled voices of those who talk about cancer. I see it in those who feverishly examine themselves for lumps or who decline to, in those so scared of getting cancer in their second breast that they're willing to cut it off, too, even when that won't help them live longer.

I find it in myself as I imagine what it would be like to get that awful diagnosis, and as I remember my agony when my daughter was diagnosed. And, if I'm honest with you, in my irrational fear that just by shining light on the cancer metaphor and writing this book about it, I will be struck with a rogue cell of my own, as if in retribution from some maleficent god of old.

A Coat Hanger and a Bag

I have a favorite image of John's cancer years. We were in Jamaica for several days together one January, about three years after his diagnosis. John and Thea had rented a villa on the beach for a few weeks and had invited Jim and me and their kids and grandchildren and, later, other relatives to visit. A winter treat.

John had begun to take the cancer in stride. He arrived in Montego Bay with a red rolling suitcase filled with his naturopathic pills: fractionated pectin, mushroom extract, green tea extract, curcumin. They were carefully counted out and packaged in individual Ziplocs for each day's consumption, an assembly line of hope.

After the bone-jarring two-and-a-half-hour car ride to the lightly populated south of the island, to a place called, appropriately, Bliss by the Sea, John got to work. The first thing on his agenda was to find a doctor who would administer the correct amount of vitamin C through an intravenous drip. He started working the phones, the neighbors, everyone he could, plotting out how he would make sure he could get his infusions.

Within an hour or so, he had it figured out. The doctor was in a town about 20 minutes away by car. He lined up a vehicle and driver to take him, set an appointment to see the doctor the next day and then arranged for similar visits for the several weeks he was to be in Jamaica.

The next day, while the rest of us lounged in the villa, sprawled in our linens over the brown wooden veranda chairs with their bright turquoise cushions, welcoming the cooling ocean breeze, off he went. He returned about an hour later, clutching an IV bag that was still attached by needle to a vein in his arm, rushed in without a word, rooted around for a coat hanger, threaded the bag onto the hanger through the hole on its top and then hung the hanger over a lamp on the wall in the eating area while he sat at the dining table until it had drained into him. A makeshift IV pole, dreamed up on the spot. He hadn't had the patience to wait it out in the doctor's office, so, as usual, he took matters into his own hands.

It was all in a day's work. It didn't faze him at all. In fact, I think he was proud of his sleuthing skills at finding the right doctor in a country he'd just arrived in. It was like landing in India and heading off to a tiny, dirt-floor village to try to make life better for people who lived there. It was the thrill of launching a new company in India in a new industry and then just seeing if it would take off. It was helping the Maasai figure out how educating their village could help people stay alive instead of dying of AIDS. It was clapping eyes on an exhausted gravel pit and envisioning a whole new way of producing food and energy and reducing greenhouse gas emissions for an entire county.

Dealing with cancer had just become part of his life. He wasn't looking for a cure any more. He was managing his melanoma — one of the most deadly of cancers — like a chronic illness, learning day by day how different cancer is from the stories we tell about it.

And this is one lesson I take from him. There was the shock of his first diagnosis of prostate cancer. Then, his second diagnosis of lethal melanoma, followed by our flailing around to assess treatments when the traditional medical system couldn't offer anything. But finally, it was his willingness to accept cancer as part of his life. To reject the idea that cancer had erased his personality, had polluted him, had reduced him to something less than he had been. He wasn't a good soldier or a valiant fighter or a trusty hero. He was simply John with cancer, doing his best. And he had things to do. Like make a garden. Change the world.

Philosopher's Stone

When I started writing this book, I didn't know if John would still be alive when I finished it. It was a story, poignantly, with an unknown end. But he is alive. He's had not a single day of illness since his diagnosis five years ago. No more tumors. No more surgeries. So far.

177

What he's had are hundreds upon hundreds of intravenous vitamin C infusions — so many that his favorite vein has collapsed and won't take the needle anymore. He was telling me recently that these days, he drinks lots of water in the hour before he shows up at Papadogianis's clinic so that the remaining veins are easier to poke. It's getting harder to find good ones. Papadogianis wonders if John has had more vitamin C flow into his blood than any other person in history. I keep reminding John to have medical assessments of his kidney function, because those organs are so often pressed into extraordinary service to get rid of the excess vitamin C and other fluids.

He's had dozens of vials of blood drawn and sent to Germany to be analyzed for the presence of circulating melanoma cells. He keeps the results on a chart he updates every five weeks when another test comes in. Because he can afford it, he also has regular, whole-body MRIs at a private clinic that search for melanoma cells that might have made their way into his organs, clumped up and made tumors. They've all been clear. The CT scan his oncologist ordered for him recently — the first in more than four years — was also clear.

So not only is he alive five years after the diagnosis, he is rudely healthy. He's lived long enough and in robust enough health that the federal Food and Drug Administration in the U.S. has approved — after rafts of clinical tests — two new drugs to treat melanoma at an advanced stage. So even if his debauched cell should form a tumor in one of his vital organs, there are two new ways for doctors to try to keep him alive. This is the man who was told that 40 per cent of patients in his situation would be dead within five years.

He has no doubt that he's happened on a course of treatment that has saved his life. To him, if it walks like a duck and quacks like a duck, it's a duck. He's taken this alternative course of treatment and so far his cancer hasn't come back. He sees a causal link between the two. In fact, he's sent many people with advanced stages of cancer to sit in the brown leather chair in Papadogianis's office in Barrie to get liquid vitamin C pumped into their blood. And they often report feeling better. Vitamin C is a powerful anti-inflammatory agent and has been shown by some small, well-conducted clinical studies to reduce the negative side effects of chemotherapy in some people, including one study of 27 ovarian cancer patients by Yan Ma and others published in 2014 in *Science Translational Medicine*. John told me about yet another acquaintance — this one had advanced colon cancer and is on chemotherapy — who was making his way to that brown chair.

Like those tumor cells that may be circulating in his body, like the metaphors that describe cancer, like the treatments doctors devise to treat it, like experiments scientists perform, John longs for replicability. He wants others to reap the benefits of what he's been through. He's based his whole life on this. The village in India, the HIV/AIDS project in Kenya, the food and energy hub in rural Ontario. He muses about bringing the Pachmann test to

Canada, of growing high-grade organic botanical pharmaceuticals to help cancer patients, of setting up a cancer center where others can experience what he has found.

The knock against that is that John's experiment is unusual even in the annals of naturopathic medicine, which is not held to all the standards of orthodox medicine: his cancer was caught early; he had no chemotherapy or radiation available as treatments; he opted for vitamin C, delivered intravenously; then he tried to check its efficacy with blood tests, the meaning of which is unclear. Not only that, but he has been on numerous other alternative therapies throughout these cancer years, including injectable mistletoe extracts, the effects of which are also unknown and unknowable. His is an uncontrolled experiment of one.

And yet the technologies to count circulating epithelial cells that John has been using might some day be the key to much more effective treatments for cancer. He's an early adopter whose years' worth of data might help others if they got into the right hands. The technology is close to being able to conduct a liquid biopsy. The blood tests are advancing so quickly that in late 2014, researchers have begun experimenting with looking into the blood for circulating bits of a cancer cell's genetic code that have been spat out as the cell died and broke open, yet another way in which peering into a living body can provide clues about the intent of that single degenerate cell and its clones.

Katharina Pachmann is investigating new ideas about

tumor cells that circulate in the body. Sometimes, she's found, an individual cell can perform as a dangerously reproductive stem cell; sometimes it can't. The ability seems to turn on and off. The mechanism is still unknown.

And circulating cancer cells might also be able to turn on and off their impulse to colonize vital organs, she says. It's unclear what triggers the switch, but it's fascinating to know it might be there, that it might be possible to lull them to sleep. This is a different way of looking at cancer than the one society has been holding onto, that of implacable tumor cells poised at all moments to attack an unsuspecting organ, every single one of which must be eradicated. It takes back an element of control and just maybe it will allow us to begin to break down our destructive cancer metaphors.

John is exploring the new frontiers of cancer therapies within the cells of his own body, at his own expense. But has he found the philosopher's stone? If I got cancer, would I do what John has done?

When I started this book, I thought that this was the most important question. Ultimately, what I've learned is that it is far messier and more complex and less certain than that. The truth is that there is sometimes no single right way to deal with cancer. Sometimes, there is an accepted medical protocol that has a result that most people can count on much of the time. That's what happened with Calista's thyroid cancer. It's not what happened with John's prostate cancer; side effects of the surgery will dog him for the rest of his life. With cancer, it's rare to find guarantees, even as we long for them. Most of the time, you just do the best you can under the circumstances.

So when we started out, I was the one wedded to the rigor of science. I was the one emitting the howl of indignation over the heavy social fallout from this metaphor that had strayed so far from the truth. I was determined to excavate the statistics, the studies, the clinical trials, trying to trace the evolution of the metaphor through time and figure out how it had gone so badly askew. It was my quest to peel back the ugly layers of this metaphor with the scalpel of knowledge.

John took another tack. Where I demanded science and certainty, he ultimately chose faith, or meaning, or perhaps narrative. Faith based on the best science available to him, to be sure, and in the absence of the existence of more closely studied options. But faith nonetheless. It was the inevitable choice for him; it's how he approaches life.

John asked me recently, rather intently, if I would advise him to quit his treatments. I would not. I'm certain he feels better doing what he is doing. But to me, there's not nearly enough evidence here to say that he's found the magic bullet that everyone should try. He's found the best answers for him, in his unique circumstances, for now.

And he has played mightily with the metaphor as he has responded to the health crisis cancer endowed him with. He has dandled it on his knee and chucked it under its chin and refused to take it seriously. He will not be bowed by shame in his diagnosis. He does not examine his conscience in the middle of the night to discern which of his sins displeased the gods. He sees his melanoma as pretty much random. Not inevitable. Possibly preventable if only we had known decades ago about the power of sunburn to pervert a skin cell. Not deserved.

But while vitamin C might be helping him in ways difficult to measure, we can never know for sure what it's doing to those melanoma cells, if, indeed, his body still has some. I can't. Papadogianis can't. Pachmann can't. John can't. And even if it happens to be killing his cells off and keeping them in check, it might not for somebody else.

I'm not sure that matters. And maybe that's the other lesson I learned from John. Maybe my quest has been not just to unpack the cancer metaphor, but also to realize that on some level, dealing with cancer must be radically personal, even theological or cosmological or philosophical. I hope that doesn't sound anti-scientific. I mean it to be a loving counterpart to some of the haranguing cancer maxims in the public discourse.

I'm thinking about the members of that First Nation in northern Manitoba I spent time with as I was waiting for John's diagnosis. They were rapt, listening to the stories their shamans told them about how their people and lands came to be. What were they here on this planet for? And why? They longed to understand. Once they knew that, they told me, they could start to live, start to move past the pain and shame they had endured. They could make choices based on what they believed about how they fit into the universe. As it was for that First Nation, so it is for all humanity.

I'm not talking about abandoning science or statistics or clinical trials, suspending one's capacity for rational thinking and embracing crank cures. Quite the opposite. I'm just wondering whether, in the end, it takes both science and faith — or cosmology or philosophy or personal narrative, or whatever you would call it — to make a whole picture. When John's Toronto oncologist told him that nothing he did would make a shred of difference, and to just go home and wait for the tumors to grow, she was badly underestimating the broad canvas that is the human spirit.

Science gives us the data and faith gives us the reason to follow the data and then, if that isn't working, to invoke the imagination, to soar beyond the numbers and surrender to the mysteries of life and death. This same impulse has driven much of medical research over the ages: dream, experiment, fail and then dream again.

COMMON, RANDOM, UNLUCKY

Maybe, in the end, the real point of this journey is to expand one's point of view. Maybe it's to realize that a good dose of scientific explanation is necessary, but it doesn't go far enough. Knowledge is power, but only to a point. Maybe in the end, it's about liberating the facts in order to rewrite the metaphor.

This is different from what Sontag asked society to do, to free disease from metaphor and see it solely as a physiological phenomenon. Like Jack Coulehan, writing in the *Yale Journal of Biology and Medicine* in 2003, I believe that patients understand their diseases in terms of metaphor whether they mean to or not. "Illness and healing are inextricably bound to narrative, meaning and metaphor," he writes. It's part of what makes us human. We tell stories; it's how we make sense of our world. And our diseases, including cancer, are part of our life's stories. We will never think only physiologically.

So, what could revised cancer metaphors look like? For one thing, they would refrain from plugging into that impossible triumvirate of inevitable, preventable and deserved. More accurate is common, random and unlucky, a trio that doesn't have the stomach punch of the current metaphor.

The messages are overblown that imply cancer is rampant, out of control, akin to a deadly virus that is sweeping the world. Cancer is actually not a "terrorist" skulking around in our society, waiting to wipe us out. We will all die, but most of us will die of something else. And if we do end up with cancer, the chances of dying of it are somewhat smaller than they were a few decades ago. Cancer is common, but it's not inevitable.

Perhaps a little context to offset the fear. The militaristic vocabulary of cancer as the implacable, pervasive enemy was developed in the middle of the last century as a marketing gambit to leverage money from individuals and the government, as Mukherjee recounts. Cancer didn't have that gloss before then. Since that time, our scientific understanding of cancer has become more nuanced. We have tracked far better the mechanism of cancer, even if we don't often know the trigger. Survival rates have increased for most cancers. Cancer rates, while still high, have actually declined in the Western world for most of the major types, adjusted for age and population growth.

But the war metaphor has, if anything, become harsher and more strident rather than more nuanced. It's worth remembering that it's being used because it's effective; it's part of a rather cynical fundraising strategy aimed at liberating dollars from your pocket. The people writing the copy for cancer fundraising campaigns are selling something, not providing accurate medical information. It's in their interests to reinforce the impossible belief system of inevitable, preventable and deserved. Part of the rewriting of the metaphor could involve holding those powerful fundraisers and others to a higher standard of intellectual honesty, forcing them to modify their vocabulary.

What about prevention, and the sister notion that if cancer should strike it represents deserved retribution? As it stands now, preventing cancer is cast as forgoing risky behavior or "suboptimal" living. It's a set of dictates, a rigid code of conduct one must follow, an exhortation to be pure in thought as well as deed. If you get cancer, the logic runs, you have not been pure enough and therefore it's your fault. But that code changes all the time according to new findings and new interpretations of old findings. (Apart from the data on tobacco.) It's almost impossible to be good enough all the time, meaning, even if you accept the code, that dodging responsibility for getting cancer is wretchedly difficult. And how much "optimal" living is enough? Is there any use living "optimally" on some fronts but "suboptimally" on others, or should one abandon all hope and dance the jig of total self-indulgence? In my own case, I'm a champion when it comes to organic broccoli and healthful walks, but I stay awake at night worrying about how much I weigh and the fact that I drink wine. Am I scuppered?

Even if one could be faithful to the code, the argument that cancer is preventable and therefore deserved if you get it breaks down badly in the science. There are 200 types of cancer and few are in our power to prevent, except those caused by tobacco and other known, avoidable, proven carcinogens. We have to accept that we cannot control the random rogue cell that might run amok in our bodies. Often, getting cancer is just bad luck. Or it's a function of advanced age. Or it means you've dodged every single other bullet life has thrown your way. It's not that you're a terrible, sinful person who has let down the whole society.

And is cancer a disease of our civilization? In a strange way, yes. The fact that our society has all but eliminated so many infectious diseases that once killed millions

— smallpox and pneumonia, for example — and has developed ways to keep people alive who have once deadly diseases — pacemakers, beta-blockers, insulin, for example — means that more people get to old age. That's when cancer is more apt to appear, because the genetic instruction book of the body's cells has more time to degrade. In the majority of cases, people who would have died young from something else in earlier eras are simply living long enough to get cancer.

It may also be that we have created a toxic world that fosters cancer, but the evidence is largely lacking. We know that industrial pollutants are common in the air and water; pesticides leave residues in food. The scientific examination of how they affect cancer rates is unsatisfactory and has been put on the back burner as investigation has focused on individual action. Our society has already set up regulatory systems to scan for carcinogenic qualities in some chemicals and is capable of banning those chemicals if they prove dangerous. To me, there is a compelling case to investigate further. If it should happen that rigorous studies show carcinogenic effects from those chemicals, we could ban or limit them. We could repair a toxic system. It's not game over.

So, taking all that into account, a few possible new cancer metaphors occur to me.

For some, it's unproductive to be told endlessly what to do. People like to make decisions. I'm thinking of a neuroscientist I once interviewed in the U.K. who explained to me that people play video games in order to experience risk. If there were only a single way to win the game, it wouldn't be fun. Decision-making is quintessentially human, he said. So, what if we were to look at the pieces of the prevention puzzle that are within our control, as if the effort were a complicated video game? We're making the best decisions we can in the moment, sometimes risking making a bad decision, but pretty safe in the knowledge that we can make a better decision later in the game. Instead of an inflexible protocol that demanded absolutes and allowed no missteps, it would be more forgiving. More human. You had French fries last night? Well, today you can choose to have a raw spinach salad. The trope of the Inquisition would recede, I think, and so might some of the anxiety.

And what if rather than preventing cancer, a fearsomely daunting task after all, the discourse were about cutting down your chances of getting it? There's something compelling about knowing you're doing your best under the circumstances. So, not a code, but a flexible recipe. Not absolutes but creativity, the joy of developing a complex and satisfying dish that you can adapt as you need to, according to the ingredients you have available.

Or perhaps a chemical experiment. Lakoff and Johnson write about one of their students at Berkeley University in California, an Iranian, who heard the expression "the solution of my problem" and envisioned a large vat of liquid compounds containing all the problems reacting with catalysts, changing all the time into new forms and new chemical formulae. In this metaphor, the problems never fully disappear; one's control over them is only partial; their reappearance is normal; each chemical reaction affects all the others in an interconnected system and also depends on all of them. If cancer were envisioned as a chemical experiment, trying to prevent it or deal with it would be a series of well-thought-out additions to the vat in an open-minded test to see what occurred, realizing that some of the reactions might be surprising. It would be an exercise in fascination and discovery.

Or what about an ecosystem? Two decades ago, in an article in the *New England Journal of Medicine*, George Annas of the Boston University Schools of Medicine and Public Health pointed to the ecologists' vocabulary of balance, limits, sustainability, conservation, responsibility for future generations. Using this metaphor might help society explore the idea of quality of life (instead of short-term winning and losing), the limits to the success of treatment, the value of planning for the long term and for the health of the whole population.

So instead of looking merely at individual risk factors and putting the blame on individuals who get sick, this metaphor would encourage looking at systems that create illness. As Annas puts it, rather than villagers setting up complex methods to save people from drowning, they would look upstream to see who was pushing them in the river in the first place and then figure out how keep people out of the water.

So, cancer as an ecosystem. Cancer as a chemistry experiment. Cancer as a creative cooking recipe, or as a complex video game. I don't mean this to be comprehensive, but simply the spark to a conversation. The point is that metaphors can evolve. We just need to give them permission.

I wonder what it would feel like if cancer were a dance, like the example of the argument Lakoff and Johnson write about in their book on metaphor. What would it feel like then? The person with cancer would be a dancer, creating art and maybe beauty and maybe life. Dances take different forms. Some are anarchic. Some dissonant. Some disruptive. Others balletic and gentle and athletic. But they are always radically personal. It's hard to feel polluted when you dance. Hard to feel as though your very self has been erased. I think John is dancing.

This is not to put an additional burden on people with cancer, a demand that they fit yet another stereotype. It is to explore how it would feel if people with cancer were seen in this way, or in another helpful way. How it might reshape the way society thinks about cancer. Not a win or a loss, but a pirouette.

Acknowledgments

Many thanks to John and Thea Patterson for opening up your journey to my scrutiny, for your kindness, wisdom and faith, and to Calista Michel for letting me write about the inner workings of your cells and for letting me tell your birth story.

Immense thanks to the Lannan Foundation for the writing fellowship in Marfa, Texas, that allowed me to bring this book to life: having time, space, a gorgeous house and a superb library made all the difference. Thanks to Lannan fellows Bill Johnston of Indiana University and Nick Turse of TomDispatch, and to Douglas Humble, Kristin Bonkemeyer and Mary Bonkemeyer of Marfa for midwifery services as the book was being born.

Thanks to early readers Marlene Sagada, Jacques Gerin, David Hallman and Connie Mitchell, and to my brilliant sister-in-law Sheela Hota-Mitchell for end-stage ministrations. The book would not have happened without support from Sally Harding, Susan Renouf, Jack David and my beloved Jim Patterson.

David Wilson and Jocelyn Bell of the *United Church Observer* gave me early encouragement and the chance to write a feature on this book's theme and also came up with the book's title, used here with their gracious permission.

Selected Bibliography

INTRODUCTION:
INEVITABLE, PREVENTABLE AND DESERVED?

Altmann, Cathy. "'To Use a Metaphor at a Time Like This Would Be Obscene': A Study of Cancer, Poetry and Metaphor." *Colloquy: Text Theory Critique* 15 (2008). artsonline.monash.edu.au/colloquy/download/colloquy_issue_fifteen/altmann.pdf.

Benedictow, Ole J. "The Black Death: The Greatest Catastrophe Ever." *History Today* 55, no. 3 (2005).

Cahill, Thomas. *Mysteries of the Middle Ages: The Rise of Feminism, Science and Art from the Cults of Catholic Europe.* New York: N.A. Talese, 2006.

Cantor, Norman F. *In the Wake of the Plague: The Black Death and the World It Made.* New York: Simon & Schuster, 2015.

Colborn, Theo, Dianne Dumanoski, and John Peterson Myers. *Our Stolen Future: Are We Threatening Our Fertility, Intelligence, and Survival? A Scientific Detective Story.* New York: Dutton, 1996.

Kelly, John. *The Great Mortality: An Intimate History of the Black Death, the Most Devastating Plague of All Time.* New York: HarperCollins, 2005.

King, R. J. B., and Mike W. Robins. *Cancer Biology.* Harlow, England: Pearson/Prentice Hall, 2006.

Lakoff, George, and Mark Johnson. *Metaphors We Live By.* Chicago: University of Chicago Press, 1980.

Mukherjee, Siddhartha. *The Emperor of All Maladies: A Biography of Cancer.* New York: Scribner, 2010.

Olson, James Stuart. *Bathsheba's Breast: Women, Cancer & History.* Baltimore: Johns Hopkins University Press, 2002.

Orenstein, Peggy. "Our Feel-Good War on Breast Cancer." *The New York Times Magazine*. April 25, 2013. nytimes.com/2013/04/28/magazine/our-feel-good-war-on-breast-cancer.html.

Peled, Ronit, Devora Carmil, Orly Siboni-Samocha, and Ilana Shoham-Vardi. "Breast Cancer, Psychological Distress and Life Events among Young Women." *BMC Cancer* 8, no. 1 (2008): 245. doi:10.1186/1471-2407-8-245.

Portschy, Pamela R., Karen M. Kuntz, and Todd M. Tuttle. "Survival Outcomes After Contralateral Prophylactic Mastectomy: A Decision Analysis." *Journal of the National Cancer Institute* 106, no. 8 (2014). doi:10.1093/jnci/dju160.

Schattner, Elaine. "The Truth about Breast Cancer and Drinking Red Wine — or Any Alcohol." *The Atlantic* (2012). theatlantic.com/health/archive/2012/01/the-truth-about-breast-cancer-and-drinking-red-wine-or-any-alcohol/251171.

ScienceDaily. sciencedaily.com.

Sontag, Susan. *AIDS and Its Metaphors*. New York: Farrar, Straus and Giroux, 1989.

Sontag, Susan. *Illness as Metaphor*. New York: Farrar, Straus and Giroux, 1978.

Stand Up to Cancer. standup2cancer.org.

Wilber, Ken. *Grace and Grit: Spirituality and Healing in the Life and Death of Treya Killam Wilber*. Boston: Shambhala, 1991.

Wilson, Kate, and Karen A. Luker. "At Home in Hospital? Interaction and Stigma in People Affected by Cancer." *Social Science & Medicine* 62, no. 7 (2006): 1616–1627. doi:10.1016/j.socscimed.2005.08.053.

Yao, Katharine, Andrew K. Stewart, David J. Winchester, and David P. Winchester. "Trends in Contralateral Prophylactic Mastectomy for Unilateral Cancer: A Report from the National Cancer

Data Base, 1998–2007." *Annals of Surgical Oncology* 17, no. 10 (2010): 2554–2562. doi:10.1245/s10434-010-1091-3.

CHAPTER 1:
PANDORA'S JAR: DISEASE AS PUNISHMENT

Benedictow, Ole J. "The Black Death: The Greatest Catastrophe Ever." *History Today* 55, no. 3 (2005).

Cahill, Thomas. *Mysteries of the Middle Ages: The Rise of Feminism, Science and Art from the Cults of Catholic Europe.* New York: N.A. Talese, 2006.

Cantor, Norman F. *In the Wake of the Plague: The Black Death and the World It Made.* New York: Simon & Schuster, 2015.

CHAPTER 2:
THE SISTERS OF FATE: IS CANCER INEVITABLE?

Jemal, A., M. M. Center, C. DeSantis, and E. M. Ward. "Global Patterns of Cancer Incidence and Mortality Rates and Trends." *Cancer Epidemiology Biomarkers & Prevention* 19, no. 8 (2010): 1893–1907. doi:10.1158/1055-9965.EPI-10-0437.

Kohler, B. A., E. Ward, B. J. McCarthy, M. J. Schymura, L. A. G. Ries, C. Eheman, A. Jemal, R. N. Anderson, U. A. Ajani, and B. K. Edwards. "Annual Report to the Nation on the Status of Cancer, 1975–2007, Featuring Tumors of the Brain and Other Nervous System." *JNCI Journal of the National Cancer Institute* 103, no. 9 (2011): 714–736. doi:10.1093/jnci/djr077.

Mukherjee, Siddhartha. *The Emperor of All Maladies: A Biography of Cancer.* New York: Scribner, 2010.

Olson, James Stuart. *Bathsheba's Breast: Women, Cancer & History.* Baltimore: Johns Hopkins University Press, 2002.

Papac, Rose J. "Origins of Cancer Therapy." *Yale Journal of Biology and Medicine* 74 (2001): 391–398.

CHAPTER 3:

BILLBOARD FOR SIN: THE FABLES OF DISEASE

Brown, John R., and John L. Thornton. "Percivall Pott (1714–1788) and Chimney Sweepers' Cancer of the Scrotum." *British Journal of Industrial Medicine* 14, no. 1 (January 1957): 68–70.

Cawthorne, Jane. "The Cure for a Cancer Cliché." Unpublished.

Chamberlain, G. "British Maternal Mortality in the 19th and Early 20th Centuries." *Journal of the Royal Society of Medicine* 99, no. 11 (2006): 559–563. doi:10.1258/jrsm.99.11.559.

Colborn, Theo, Dianne Dumanoski, and John Peterson Myers. *Our Stolen Future: Are We Threatening Our Fertility, Intelligence and Survival? A Scientific Detective Story.* New York: Dutton, 1996.

Dahl, Alv A. "Link between Personality and Cancer." *Future Oncology* 6, no. 5 (May 2010).

Jokela, M., G. D. Batty, T. Hintsa, M. Elovainio, C. Hakulinen, and M. Kivimäki. "Is Personality Associated with Cancer Incidence and Mortality? An Individual-Participant Meta-Analysis of 2156 Incident Cancer Cases among 42,843 Men and Women." *British Journal of Cancer* 110, no. 7 (2014): 1820–1824. doi:10.1038/bjc.2014.58.

Lemogne, C., S. M. Consoli, B. Geoffroy-Perez, M. Coeuret-Pellicer, H. Nabi, M. Melchior, F. Limosin, M. Zins, P. Ducimetière, M. Goldberg, and S. Cordier. "Personality and the Risk of Cancer: A 16-Year Follow-Up Study of the GAZEL Cohort." *Psychosomatic Medicine* 75, no. 3 (2013): 262–271. doi:10.1097/PSY.0b013e31828b5366.

"METABRIC." British Columbia Cancer Agency, Department of

Molecular Oncology. Accessed April 7, 2015. molonc.bccrc.ca/
aparicio-lab/research/metabric.

Parkin, D. M., L. Boyd, and L. C. Walker. "The Fraction of Cancer
Attributable to Lifestyle and Environmental Factors in the
UK in 2010." *British Journal of Cancer* 105 (2011): S77-81.
doi:10.1038/bjc.2011.489.

Reuben, Suzanne H. *Reducing Environmental Cancer Risk: What We
Can Do Now.* Report. 2008–2009 Annual Report, President's
Cancer Panel. U.S. Dept. of Health and Human Services,
National Institutes of Health, National Cancer Institute, April,
2010. deainfo.nci.nih.gov/advisory/pcp/annualReports/
pcp08-09rpt/PCP_Report_08-09_508.pdf.

Rosch, Paul J. "Stress and Cancer: A Disease of Adaptation?" In
Cancer, Stress, and Death, edited by S. B. Day, 187–212. New
York: Plenum Medical Book, 1979. doi:10.1007/978-1-4684-
3459-0_18.

Tăut, Diana. "Is It Ethical to Advise People to 'Fight' Cancer?" *The
European Health Psychologist* 16, no. 3 (June 2014): 107–110.

Wilber, Ken. *Grace and Grit: Spirituality and Healing in the Life and
Death of Treya Killam Wilber.* Boston: Shambhala, 1991.

CHAPTER 4:
THE HARUSPEX: DEFYING THE DREAD

Cabanillas, Fernando. "Vitamin C and Cancer: What Can We
Conclude — 1,609 Patients and 33 Years Later?" *Puerto Rico
Health Sciences Journal* 29, no. 3 (September 2010): 215–217.

Cameron, Ewan, and Linus Pauling. *Cancer and Vitamin C: A
Discussion of the Nature, Causes, Prevention, and Treatment of
Cancer with Special Reference to the Value of Vitamin C.* Menlo Park,
CA: Linus Pauling Institute of Science and Medicine, 1979.

Cullen, Joseph J., Douglas R. Spitz, and Garry R. Buettner. "Comment on 'Pharmacologic Ascorbate Synergizes with Gemcitabine in Pre-Clinical Models of Pancreatic Cancer' i.e. All We Are Saying Is Give C a Chance." *Free Radical Biology and Medicine* 50, no. 12 (June 2011): 1726–1727. doi: 10.1016/j.freeradbiomed.2011.03.030.

DeVita, V. T., and E. Chu. "A History of Cancer Chemotherapy." *Cancer Research* 68, no. 21 (2008): 8643–8653. doi:10.1158/0008-5472.CAN-07-6611.

Frei, Baltz, and Stephen Lawson. "Vitamin C and Cancer Revisited." *Proceedings of the National Academy of Sciences* 105, no. 32 (August 12, 2008): 11037–11038. doi:10.1073/pnas.0806433105.

Grasso, Carole, Marie-Sophie Fabre, Sarah V. Collis, M. Leticia Castro, Cameron S. Field, Nanette Schleich, Melanie J. McConnell, and Patries M. Herst. "Pharmacological Doses of Daily Ascorbate Protect Tumors from Radiation Damage after a Single Dose of Radiation in an Intracranial Mouse Glioma Model." *Frontiers in Oncology* 4 (December 15, 2014). doi:10.3389/fonc.2014.00356.

Heaney, M. L., J. R. Gardner, N. Karasavvas, D. W. Golde, D. A. Scheinberg, E. A. Smith, and O. A. O'Connor. "Vitamin C Antagonizes the Cytotoxic Effects of Antineoplastic Drugs." *Cancer Research* 68, no. 19 (2008): 8031–8038. doi:10.1158/0008-5472.CAN-08-1490.

Hoffer, L. J., M. Levine, S. Assouline, D. Melnychuk, S. J. Padayatty, K. Rosadiuk, C. Rousseau, L. Robitaille, and W. H. Miller. "Phase I Clinical Trial of I.V. Ascorbic Acid in Advanced Malignancy." *Annals of Oncology* 19, no. 11 (2008): 1969–1974. doi:10.1093/annonc/mdn377.

Levine, M., S. J. Padayatty, and M. G. Espey. "Vitamin C: A Concentration-Function Approach Yields Pharmacology and Therapeutic Discoveries." *Advances in Nutrition: An International Review Journal* 2, no. 2 (2011): 78–88. doi:10.3945/an.110.000109.

Luengo-Fernandez, Ramon, Jose Leal, Alastair Gray, and Richard Sullivan. "Economic Burden of Cancer across the European Union: A Population-Based Cost Analysis." *The Lancet Oncology* 14, no. 12 (2013): 1165–1174. doi:10.1016/S1470-2045(13)70442-X.

Ma, Y., J. Chapman, M. Levine, K. Polireddy, J. Drisko, and Q. Chen. "High-Dose Parenteral Ascorbate Enhanced Chemosensitivity of Ovarian Cancer and Reduced Toxicity of Chemotherapy." *Science Translational Medicine* 6, no. 222 (2014): 222ra18. doi:10.1126/scitranslmed.3007154.

McConnell, M. J., and P. M. Herst. "Ascorbate Combination Therapy: New Tool in the Anticancer Toolbox?" *Science Translational Medicine* 6, no. 222 (2014): 222fs6. doi:10.1126/scitranslmed.3008488.

Michelakis, E. D., G. Sutendra, P. Dromparis, L. Webster, A. Haromy, E. Niven, C. Maguire, T. L. Gammer, J. R. Mackey, D. Fulton, B. Abdulkarim, M. S. McMurtry, and K. C. Petruk. "Metabolic Modulation of Glioblastoma with Dichloroacetate." *Science Translational Medicine* 2, no. 31 (2010): 31ra34. doi:10.1126/scitranslmed.3000677.

Michelakis, E. D., L. Webster, and J. R. Mackey. "Dichloroacetate as a Potential Metabolic-targeting Therapy for Cancer." *British Journal of Cancer* 99 (2008): 989–994. doi:10.1038/sj.bjc.6604554.

Moertel, Charles G., Thomas R. Fleming, Edward T. Greagan, Joseph Rubin, Michael J. O'Connell, and Matthew M. Ames. "High-Dose Vitamin C versus Placebo in the Treatment of Patients with Advanced Cancer Who Have Had No Prior Chemotherapy: A Randomized Double-Blind Comparison."

The New England Journal of Medicine 312, no. 3 (January 17, 1985): 137–141.

Moss, Ralph. Cancer Decisions: The Moss Reports, The Trusted Source for Cancer News and Opinion. Accessed April 8, 2015. cancerdecisions.com.

Ohno, Satoshi, Yumiko Ohno, Nobutaka Suzuki, Gen-Ichiro Soma, and Masaki Inoue. "High-Dose Vitamin C (Ascorbic Acid) Therapy in the Treatment of Patients with Advanced Cancer." *Anticancer Research* 29 (2009): 809–816.

Ostermann, Thomas, Christa Raak, and Arndt Büssing. "Survival of Cancer Patients Treated with Mistletoe Extract (Iscador): A Systematic Literature Review." *BMC Cancer* 9, no. 1 (2009): 451. doi:10.1186/1471-2407-9-451.

Padayatty, Sebastian J., Hugh D. Riordan, Stephen M. Hewitt, Arie Katz, John Hoffer, and Mark Levine. "Intravenously Administered Vitamin C as Cancer Therapy: Three Cases." *Canadian Medical Association Journal* 174, no. 7 (2006): 937–942. doi:10.1503/cmaj.050346.

Padayatty, Sebastian J., and Mark Levine. "New Insights into the Physiology and Pharmacology of Vitamin C." *Canadian Medical Association Journal* 164, no. 3 (February 6, 2001): 353–355.

Parrow, Nermi L., Jonathan A. Leshin, and Mark Levine. "Parenteral Ascorbate as a Cancer Therapeutic: A Reassessment Based on Pharmacokinetics." *Antioxidants & Redox Signaling* 19, no. 17 (2013): 2141–2156. doi:10.1089/ars.2013.5372.

Welsh, J. L., B. A. Wagner, T. J. Van'T Erve, P. S. Zehr, D. J. Berg, T. R. Halfdanarson, N. S. Yee, K. L. Bodeker, J. Du, L. J. Roberts, J. Drisko, M. Levine, G. R. Buettner, and J. J. Cullen. "Pharmacological Ascorbate with Gemcitabine for the Control of Metastatic and Node-Positive Pancreatic Cancer (PACMAN): Results from a Phase I Clinical Trial." *Cancer Chemotherapy and*

Pharmacology 71, no. 3 (2013): 765–775. doi:10.1007/ s00280-013-2070-8.

CHAPTER 5:

LIQUID BIOPSY: THE IMAGINATION OF CANCER

Alix-Panabières, Catherine, and Klaus Pantel. "Challenges in Circulating Tumor Cell Research." *Nature Reviews Cancer* 14 (July 31, 2014): 623–631. doi:10.1038/nrc3820.

Blue Cross of Idaho. "Detection of Circulating Tumor Cells in the Management of Patients with Cancer." Medical Policy 2.04.37, revised May 2013. bcidaho.com/providers/medical_policies/ med/mp_20437.asp.

Cristofanilli, M., and S. Braun. "Circulating Tumor Cells Revisited." *JAMA: The Journal of the American Medical Association* 303, no. 11 (2010): 1092–1093. doi:10.1001/jama.2010.292.

Cristofanilli, M., J. Reuben, and J. Uhr. "Circulating Tumor Cells in Breast Cancer: Fiction or Reality?" *Journal of Clinical Oncology* 26, no. 21 (2008): 3656–3657. doi:10.1200/ JCO.2008.18.0356.

Dong, Yi, Alison M. Skelley, Keith D. Merdek, Kam M. Sprott, Chunsheng Jiang, William E. Pierceall, Jessie Lin, Michael Stocum, Walter P. Carney, and Denis A. Smirnov. "Micro-fluidics and Circulating Tumor Cells." *The Journal of Molecular Diagnostics* 15, no. 2 (2013): 149–157. doi:10.1016/j .jmoldx.2012.09.004.

Freeman, James B., Elin S. Gray, Michael Millward, Robert Pearce, and Melanie Ziman. "Evidence of a Multi-Marker Immuno-magnetic Enrichment Assay for the Quantification of Circu-lating Melanoma Cells." *Journal of Translational Medicine* 10 (2012). doi:10.1186/1479-5876-10-192.

Hong, Bin. "Detecting Circulating Tumor Cells: Current
Challenges and New Trends." *Theranostics* 3, no. 6 (2013):
377–394. doi:10.7150/thno.5195.

Hoshimoto, Sojun, Tatsushi Shingai, Donald L. Morton, Christine
Kuo, Mark B. Faries, Kelly Chong, David Elashoff, He-Jing
Wang, Robert M. Elashoff, and Dave S.B. Hoon. "Association
Between Circulating Tumor Cells and Prognosis in Patients
with Stage III Melanoma with Sentinel Lymph Node Metastasis
in a Phase III International Multicenter Trial." *Journal of
Clinical Oncology* 30, no. 31 (November 1, 2012): 3819–3826.
doi:10.1200/jco.2011.40.0887.

Jin, Chao, Sarah M. McFaul, Simon P. Duffy, Xiaoyan Deng,
Peyman Tavassoli, Peter C. Black, and Hongshen Ma.
"Technologies for Label-Free Separation of Circulating Tumor
Cells: From Historical Foundations to Recent Developments."
Lab on a Chip 14, no. 1 (2013): 32. doi:10.1039/c3lc50625h.

Lucci, Anthony, Carolyn S. Hall, Ashutosh K. Lodhi, Anirban
Bhattacharyya, Amber E. Anderson, Lianchun Xiao, Isabelle
Bedrosian, Henry M. Kuerer, and Savitri Krishnamurthy.
"Circulating Tumor Cells in Non-Metastatic Breast Cancer:
A Prospective Study." *The Lancet Oncology* 13, no. 7 (2012):
688–695. doi:10.1016/S1470-2045(12)70209-7.

Maheswaran, Shyamala, and Daniel A. Haber. "Circulating Tumor
Cells: A Window into Cancer Biology and Metastasis." *Current
Opinion in Genetics & Development* 20, no. 1 (2010): 96–99.
doi:10.1016/j.gde.2009.12.002.

Millner, Lori M., Mark W. Linder, and Roland Valdes, Jr. "Circulating Tumor Cells: A Review of Present Methods and the Need
to Identify Heterogeneous Phenotypes." *Annals of Clinical &
Laboratory Science* 43, no. 3 (2013).

Nezos, Andrianos, Pavlos Msaouel, Nikolaos Pissimissis, Peter

Lembessis, Antigone Sourla, Athanasios Armakolas, Helen Gogas, Alexandros J. Stratigos, Andreas D. Datsambas, and Michael Koutsilieris. "Methods of Detection of Circulating Melanoma Cells: A Comparative Review." *Cancer Treatment Reviews* 37 (2011): 284–290. doi:10.1016/j.ctrv.2010.10.002.

Pantel, K., and C. Alix-Panabières. "Real-time Liquid Biopsy in Cancer Patients: Fact or Fiction?" *Cancer Research* 73, no. 21 (2013): 6384-6388. doi:10.1158/0008-5472.CAN-13-2030.

Parkinson, David R., Nicholas Dracopoli, Brenda Gumbs Petty, Carolyn Compton, Massimo Cristofanilli, Albert Deisseroth, Daniel F. Hayes, Gordon Kapke, Prasanna Kumar, Jerry S. H. Lee, Minetta C. Liu, Robert McCormack, Stanislaw Mikulski, Larry Nagahara, Klaus Pantel, Sonia Pearson-White, Elizabeth A. Punnoose, Lori T. Roadcap, Andrew E. Schade, Howard I. Scher, Caroline C. Sigman, and Gary J. Kelloff. "Considerations in the Development of Circulating Tumor Cell Technology for Clinical Use." *Journal of Translational Medicine* 10, no. 1 (2012): 138. doi:10.1186/1479-5876-10-138.

Pizon, M., D. Zimon, S. Carl, U. Pachmann, K. Pachmann, and O. Camara. "Heterogeneity of Circulating Epithelial Tumor Cells from Individual Patients with Respect to Expression Profiles and Clonal Growth (Sphere Formation) in Breast Cancer." *Ecancermedicalscience* 7 (August 23, 2013). doi:10.3332/ecancer.2013.343.

Steen, Shawn, John Nemunaitis, Tammy Fisher, and Joseph Kuhn. "Circulating Tumor Cells in Melanoma: A Review of the Literature and Description of a Novel Techique." *Baylor University Medical Center Proceedings* 21, no. 2 (2008): 127–132.

Swaby, Ramona F., and Massimo Cristofanilli. "Circulating Tumor Cells in Breast Cancer: A Tool Whose Time Has Come of Age." *BMC Medicine* 9, no. 1 (2011): 43. doi:10.1186/1741-7015-9-43.

Uhr, J. "Response to Dr. Pachmann. Re: Circulating Tumor Cells in Patients with Breast Cancer Dormancy." *Clinical Cancer Research* 11, no. 5 (2005): 5657.

Yu, M., S. Stott, M. Toner, S. Maheswaran, and D. A. Haber. "Circulating Tumor Cells: Approaches to Isolation and Characterization." *The Journal of Cell Biology* 192, no. 3 (2011): 373–382. doi:10.1083/jcb.201010021.

Zhang, L., S. Riethdorf, G. Wu, T. Wang, K. Yang, G. Peng, J. Liu, and K. Pantel. "Meta-Analysis of the Prognostic Value of Circulating Tumor Cells in Breast Cancer." *Clinical Cancer Research* 18, no. 20 (2012): 5701–5710. doi:10.1158/1078-0432.CCR-12-1587.

CHAPTER 7:
REWRITING THE METAPHOR

Annas, George J. "Reframing the Debate on Health Care Reform by Replacing Our Metaphors." *New England Journal of Medicine* 332, no. 11 (1995): 744–747.

Coulehan, Jack. "Metaphor and Medicine: Narrative in Clinical Practice." *Yale Journal of Biology and Medicine* 76 (2003): 87–95.

Hauser, David J., and Norbert Schwarz. "The War on Prevention: Bellicose Cancer Metaphors Hurt (Some) Prevention Intentions." *Personality and Social Psychology Bulletin.* Accessed October 28, 2014. doi:10.1177/0146167214557006.

Lakoff, George, and Mark Johnson. *Metaphors We Live By.* Chicago: University of Chicago Press, 1980.

Ma, Y., J. Chapman, M. Levine, K. Polireddy, J. Drisko, and Q. Chen. "High-Dose Parenteral Ascorbate Enhanced Chemosensitivity of Ovarian Cancer and Reduced Toxicity of Chemotherapy." *Science Translational Medicine* 6, no. 222 (2014): 222ra18. doi:10.1126/scitranslmed.3007154.

Penson, R. T. "Cancer as Metaphor." *The Oncologist* 9, no. 6 (2004): 708–716. doi:10.1634/theoncologist.9-6-708.

Stand Up to Cancer. standup2cancer.org.

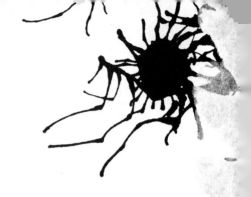

Get the eBook FREE!

At ECW Press, we want you to enjoy this book in whatever
format you like, whenever you like. Leave your print book at
home and take the eBook to go! Purchase the print edition
and receive the eBook free. Just send an email to
ebook@ecwpress.com and include:

- the book title
- the name of the store where you purchased it
- your receipt number
- your preference of file type: PDF or ePub?

A real person will respond to your email with your eBook
attached. Thank you for supporting an independently owned
Canadian publisher with your purchase!